# CLIMBING THE MOUNTAIN

# CLIMBING
## THE
# MOUNTAIN

Stories of Hope and Healing
after Stroke and Brain Injury

EDITED BY

Candis Fancher, Lindsey McDivitt,
and Jacquelyn B. Fletcher

Fairview Press
Minneapolis

Published by Fairview Press, 2450 Riverside Avenue, Minneapolis, MN 55454. Fairview Press is a division of Fairview Health Services, a community-focused health system affiliated with the University of Minnesota and providing a complete range of services, from the prevention of illness and injury to care for the most complex medical conditions. For a free current catalog of Fairview Press books, please call toll-free 1-800-544-8207, or visit our website at www. fairviewpress.org.

**Library of Congress Cataloging-in-Publication Data**
Climbing the mountain : stories of hope and healing after stroke and brain injury / edited by Candis Fancher, Lindsey McDivitt, and Jacquelyn B. Fletcher.
    p. cm.
Includes bibliographical references.
ISBN-13: 978-1-57749-192-7 (pbk. : alk. paper)
ISBN-10: 1-57749-192-0 (pbk. : alk. paper)
I. Fancher, Candis, 1950- II. McDivitt, Lindsey, 1955- III. Fletcher, Jacquelyn B., 1972-
RC388.5 .C57
362.196'8100922--dc22
                2009004722

Text design: Dorie McClelland, Spring Book Design

To the brave stroke thrivers and their families
who contributed to this anthology
and to the readers
who will benefit from their courage.

# Contents

## Coping Tips

Embrace all aspects of healing.  9  •  Trust others.  14  •  Volunteer
and advocate for others.  17  •  Challenge yourself to grow through the
frustrating times.  21  •  Choose positive words to describe your new
life.  28  •  Consider a different kind of work.  30  •  Make a word list to
practice writing.  36  •  Save your energy and spend it wisely.  39
Recovery is not a race.  55  •  Learn relaxation techniques.  58
Persistence pays off.  61  •  Grieve your losses and move forward.
66  •  Write your own story.  71  •  Read, talk, write.  75  •  Make
communication easier.  79  •  You can control your attitude.  53  •  Use a
variety of strategies to communicate.  83  •  Laugh for your health.  85
Find a new way to do what you love.  88  •  Sing to bring harmony to the
heart and strength to the body.  88  •  Use your experience to help others.
91  •  Know the signs of depression.  95  •  Discover ways you can stay
active.  98  •  Work together.  102  •  You are still the same person.  105
To improve fluency, talk about your life experiences.  107
Understand the changed brain.  113  •  Get the most you can out of rehab.
117  •  Read aloud to an audience.  122  •  Denial slows recovery.  124
Rehab is ongoing.  128  •  Find creative ways to express yourself.  134
Learn to let go.  137  •  Use your whole body.  137  •  Peer visitors offer
support to new stroke survivors.  139  •  Accept help.  143  •  Rest is
essential to the recovery process.  147  •  Reduce stress to enhance your
health.  151  •  Help a loved one with aphasia.  155  •  The ABCs of Living
with Communication Challenges.  156  •  Manage everyday life with
simple tools.  159  •  Your memory can improve with practice.  162
Carepartners also need to care for themselves.  165  •  Exercise is good for
both the body and the brain.  168  •  Don't spend time on things you can't
change.  171  •  Know the warning signs of stroke.  175  •  Use whatever
helps you.  173  •  Be honest with yourself and others.  183
Turn fear into freedom.  186  •  Don't drive after a brain injury until you
know it's safe.  192

**Medical information**

# Preface

Use this book as best fits your particular situation and needs as a stroke survivor. You may want to read the stories slowly, one at a time, over many weeks, savoring the sips of insight, advice, and encouragement each story offers. Or you may want to read the entire book in one big gulp and digest it all at once.

A word of caution: these stories may have a powerful impact on you. However, acknowledging and working through your emotions can help you heal.

If, for physical, cognitive, or emotional reasons, you find it difficult to read these stories, share the book with family, friends, and carepartners so that they can better understand what you are going through and how they can help you. Later, as you progress in your recovery process, you can read and discuss these stories with your loved ones. You may want to share your personal story with others as well. Think of this book as your own virtual support group and be assured that you are not alone as you climb the mountain to recovery.

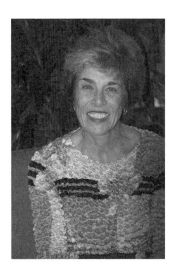

# Introduction

*by* Candis Fancher

Helen Keller once said, "Life is either a daring adventure or nothing." Recovery from stroke or brain injury takes perseverance, patience, and the ability to hold on to a *rope of hope*. In my 35 years as a speech-language pathologist, my patients have taught me many life lessons. Cheering them on as they grow through loss and grief has been a privilege to experience.

Among the pictures that hang in my office is one of a jagged mountaintop aglow in the rising sun. "Climbing the mountain" is a metaphor I often use to describe the arduous recovery process. Sometimes, when climbing a mountain, you quickly ascend steep slopes. Other times you level out over plateaus. And, occasionally, you slip down into a valley or have to backtrack before you can move ahead. Reaching the peak requires endurance, courage, and determination.

The changed brain after stroke or brain injury is a strange and unwelcome visitor to the survivor and family members. A changed brain calls for role transitions, extra effort, sacrifice, and discipline. The question I'm most frequently asked at treatment onset is, "When will my brain be normal again?" Honestly I must acknowledge that the brain will be forever different—still beautiful and full of possibilities, but changed. The brain must re-route information around the damaged area and receive information from other pathways. Sometimes the pathways are unfamiliar or less efficient. Through diligent practice, progress can occur. Accepting the new brain is the beginning step on the lifelong road to recovery. It is not a smooth walk up the mountain.

Some stories are written by family members in honor of their loved ones. Many of the writers have experienced strokes or brain injuries that have left them with aphasia. "Aphasia" refers to difficulty in any or all of the following areas: listening, reading, talking, writing, concentrating, and remembering. These writers are some of the most creative people I know, because they have discovered how to grow through pain and achieve their goals despite the barriers.

During the therapeutic process, it is possible for amazing transformations in communication and cognitive abilities to occur. To experience how simple therapeutic tips and strategies can enhance a patient's ability to unlock mental blocks and maximize brain potential is the joy of my professional journey. Some patients have returned to work despite all odds. Some have developed new interests and hobbies. Some have written and shared their personal stories to encourage and uplift others. And some have received intensive training to become peer visitors. Most, in one way or another, have become avid advocates for other stroke survivors and for their communities at large. These "stroke thrivers" have become my heroes, mentors, and friends because we have shared a crisis and grown to love each other through the recovery and self-discovery process.

My mom, Bonnie, was a stroke survivor. Her compromised stamina and limited speech eventually resolved into fluent speech because *she never gave up!* Although she chose not to drive after her stroke, she willingly jumped into a car and rode hundreds of miles to cheer on her grandchildren in their sporting events. In 2007, the year she turned 80, she walked with her grandchild down the aisle on his wedding day, looking radiant. Only a few hours before a heart attack claimed her life, she rode her stationary bike three miles, baked a double batch of bran muffins, and told each of her four children how much she loved them and that she would see them on Thanksgiving. *That's what quality of life looks like:* living with gusto and tenacity while overcoming obstacles to reach the mountaintop.

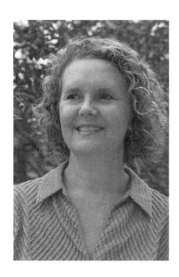

# Become a Thriver

*by* Lindsey McDivitt

Our stroke program staff love nothing more than seeing a survivor
of stroke or brain injury push through the darkness and into the
warm glow of a new life. The difference between surviving and truly
thriving is the realization that your life after stroke and brain injury
is rich with possibilities: new goals, new relationships, and satisfying
new challenges. It is our profound wish that in reading the stories
collected in this book you will, like Holly Noelle in her story "7 Out
of 10," come to know yourself to be whole and capable of joy and
growth in every area of your life.

Our stroke center staff reach out to survivors with many forms
of education and support. We believe strongly that a powerful
and healing energy is generated when survivors come together. To
facilitate a gathering of survivors we created the Stroke Showcase,
an event called "inspirational" by the audience and "a little scary" by
the participants. The courage and creativity of survivors who read
their stories on stage reinforced our resolve to share their hard-won
insights with you, along with our own very best strategies and tips

for successful recovery from stroke and brain injury.

On the evening of the Stroke Showcase, more than 100 people came together in our largest lecture hall. Tension was high as the audience of survivors and their families settled into their seats, many having never been at a gathering with other survivors. The buzz in the large room built with conversations shared over a buffet dinner. The storytellers paced or sat quietly. Tiffany, at 26 the youngest survivor, stood at the back of the room wondering, "*Why* did I agree to speak tonight?"

But when the lights dimmed and, one by one, survivors stood at the podium facing the hushed crowd, magic blossomed. Twice Tiffany conquered tears in order to finish her story of recovery from aphasia. The audience shared in her feelings of triumph. John, his wife, Linda, and their carepartner, Deondray, shared the richness gained in their special relationships. And Anna courageously acknowledged the necessary next step she would take to grieve her losses and move on.

Everyone stood a little taller that evening. The tenacity and creativity of the survivors who shared their stories struck a chord with those listening, swelling into a tremendous sense of collective pride.

Fact: A life turned upside down after stroke or brain injury often transforms into a "new normal" as the pieces fall into new patterns. Another fact: This new life can be both satisfying and joyful when you invite other people in.

Story after story demonstrated that, while the formula for success may differ somewhat for each survivor, shared insights and knowledge can make the difference between thriving and not thriving. Hearing others tell their personal stories soothes and inspires as few things can. It is our hope that these stories will serve as a lifeline to readers who most need it.

Sadly, some survivors lack community resources or access to them. Others seem to avoid the very interactions with other survivors that can be so helpful. There is too often a sense that "those people aren't like me." Many people are concerned that contact with other survivors will be depressing or require sharing of personal information. Doctors, therapists, and family members may even discourage attendance at support groups for many of the same misguided reasons.

But we've discovered that every interaction at a stroke class or group sparks new energy for the journey. We begin with daily hospital visits to patients by our peer visitors. Health care providers appreciate how the peer visitors reinforce their teachings about recovery and prevention. Meeting another stroke survivor who is obviously thriving also seems to forge a link that eventually helps draw survivors to groups and classes later in the recovery process.

"A hallmark of our program is the caring network of support that begins during the hospital stay, continues through rehabilitation, and doesn't end when a survivor goes out into the community," says Marnee Shepard, manager of the Fairview Stroke Program. "As a physical therapist, I would sense the fear as I was congratulating survivors on their successful completion of rehab therapy. I felt I was turning them out to follow an unknown and lonely path. They had completed their first course of rehabilitation but were still far removed from their original life path."

Collaboration between the Stroke Program and the Rehabilitation Department at Fairview Southdale Hospital provides survivors with the resources to continue on their journey without feeling that they have to do it alone. A series of four StrokeWise classes is designed to meet their needs six to 12 months after the event. Stroke Thrivers is a monthly support group that is part discussion and part lecture. Other collaborative efforts include the aphasia conversation group known as "Life in Bloom," our unique Tai Chi exercise program, and support for carepartners.

Education and the camaraderie of peers, combined with rehabilitation, can give survivors a powerful sense of confidence. Nancy Wells, Rehabilitation Director, describes Fairview Southdale Hospital's rehab philosophy as follows: "Traditionally, rehabilitation is thought of as a way to restore one's good health—to work with a physical therapist, occupational therapist, or speech-language pathologist for help in restoring capacity and function. Our team takes this one step further. We view survivors as individuals with unique needs, beliefs, and abilities. Our clients become part of our 'family.' In learning our survivor's desires and hopes, we can establish a trusting and meaningful relationship and work together with them on the road to successful healing."

In this book, our "family" of survivors offers their stories to help you with your own story of surviving and thriving after stroke or brain injury. You'll read about people who have experienced powerful breakthroughs, worked through emotional challenges, forged new relationships, found interesting new volunteer jobs, and shared helpful strategies for living with a changed brain. Above all, you'll learn from these pages what we discovered the night of our Stroke Showcase—that no matter how you may be struggling with the changes that have occurred in your life, you are not alone.

Courage doesn't always roar.
Sometimes courage is the quiet voice
at the end of the day saying,
"I will try again tomorrow."

MARY ANNE RADMACHER

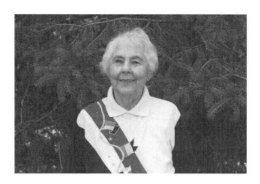

# A Special Christmas Greeting to All

*by* Renee

Renee's Christmas letter contains spelling errors, but the message is no less poignant. With this letter Renee let those she cares about know how she was doing with humor and honesty. Your family and friends want to hear from you. Isolating yourself from the people who love you can lead to serious depression. The important thing is connection, not perfection.

Please don't expect to read my usual, utterly charming Christmas message this year. Since my stroke left me with the ability to write but not to read, some of my greeting leafes some choice dialect. I am so eager to share my progress at re-learning to read, that I may not get everything quite right. Can you reak it?

I do want you to know that I am alive and well (well sort of), a little battered and missing some parts, but with God's help and a little reorganuzatuib, we'll get it together. I have been chopped and stitcged, bent to fit, and stretched with revised language skills. And eyes were added that I didn't know I had, but I'm ready for a new beginning.

Blessings on all those who helped me along the way and yet to come. How can one person become so dependent on so many? Remind me to be more understanding of uthers in the puture. Here me now: I am grateful for the joy of greeting another new day, for the memories of old Christmases, and the toucg of your many upcomg holiday greetings.

I apppologize to y oo who did not learn of my misfourtun last summer and wish for you a special absentee blessing.

A heartfelt Christmas greeing to all.

God Bless!

I hope every one's greeting has arrived because it means thn that; you have been wished a Merry Christmss and have helped me to read again—my next year's meery Christmas.

*Renée*

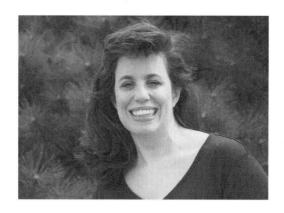

# 7 Out of 10

*by* Holly Noelle

Candis leans across the table and says, "Write a sentence using the word 'cat' in it." I think for a while and then write: "The cat eats food." "Very good," says Candis, beaming. I don't think it's very good. I think it's actually terrible. I had wanted to write about a mouse being eaten, but "The cat eats mouse" sentence I initially came up with wasn't right and I didn't know how to fix it. So I did the big switch: simple words for harder ones. Actually I had wanted to write about a cat being stalked by a psychotic mouse with delusions of grandeur. I had an Alfred Hitchcock vision in my mind, but setting the scene with sinister shadows was a little bit too advanced for me. After all, I can't even remember the plural of mouse.

I am 35 years old, and I had a stroke last year. This is why I sit across from Candis, my speech therapist, three times a week, trying to learn to speak, write, read, and even listen the right way. Having a stroke is like jumping down the rabbit hole in *Alice in Wonderland*. In one second you are in a really crazy place, trapped by your own brain. You still have far-reaching thoughts, dreams, imagination, and humor, but no way to express them. They tell me speech therapy might be the only way to get back to where I was. I have lots of doubts about that; mostly, I think I will be stuck here forever: Alice in Strokeland.

**"In one second you are in a really crazy place, trapped by your own brain. You still have far-reaching thoughts, dreams, imagination, and humor, but no way to express them. "**

I keep writing basic sentences with Candis, including one word of her choosing:

> garden
>
> rent
>
> funny
>
> mother

She is big on praise. Even my sentence "My mother is nuts" gets applause. Candis is endlessly supportive and encouraging; I get compliments galore. I ab-so-lute-ly hate it. I hate it because I don't deserve it. I can't do anything right. I make mistakes all the time. I'm tired. I want to give up.

Weeks later I am writing paragraphs. Candis gives me her assignment: "Here are six words, and I want you to include them in a paragraph."

> sun
>
> water
>
> grass
>
> buffalo
>
> wind
>
> mermaid

So much for describing a "home on the range" scene. Where did the freaking mermaid come from? I might have had a stroke, but I know that there are no mermaids on the range. The broad is out to get me.

I want to describe a mermaid eating buffalo burgers with the sun slanting through the water, and sea grass gently waving nearby, mimicking the wind—kind of like "The Little Mermaid Goes to The Hard Rock Cafe, Bermuda Triangle"—but once again I am missing all the words to put it together. I wonder if I can get away with a "Home on the Range" scene and have the buffalo eat the mermaid. Do I have to explain where the mermaid came from? Maybe a drug-induced hallucination from the buffalo smoking too much prairie grass. And then the buffalo spits out the scales, leaving his mouth a bloody mess. It will be a scathing commentary of illegal drugs as escapism. No, no, no—it will be blood as a symbolic link between reality and imagination. Or it could be the rich and previous unknown life of buffalo intellectualism: the alienation, the drama, and the secret life of b-b-b-buffalo. Oh, I am never going to be able to do this.

I stumble through it, using easy words and simple plots instead, throwing out my wild imaginings. There is always another assignment to tackle. The days I don't see Candis, I have homework. Doesn't she know I'm not going to get better? Apparently not; she won't give up on me. She is not a speech therapist; she is a speech *terrorist*.

"Write a paragraph using 12 unrelated words."

"Write a story of your own choosing."

"Write on demand."

I handle each assignment, struggling with the writing, and even more so with the compliments she lavishes on me.

"Holly, you are a powerful writer," Candis says seriously.

'Yeah, right,' I think and roll my eyes.

Another day she declares, "Holly, you have a great talent."

I mutter under my breath, "I bet you say that to all of your students."

"You don't need to learn to write." Candis the Complimenter is at it again. "You already know." I sigh heavily and think, "Then why are you torturing me with all these writing assignments?"

Candis now has a new trick. She makes me read my assignments out loud and then rate them. She thinks she will trick me into acknowledging my progress and success. I thwart her every chance I get. Everything I write is 7 out of 10. I truly believe it, so it is easy. All I can see are the faults in my pieces: the trite themes, the gaps in structure, and the sad lack of descriptive language. Oh, it's not terrible. It's just . . . okay. Not great—but . . . well, okay. It could be a lot better, that's for sure.

Candis keeps trying and I keep fighting. This goes on for some time.

"How was your homework sheet?"

"7 out of 10."

"How was your on-demand paragraph??

"7 out of 10."

"How was your pronoun-writing exercise?"

"7 out of 10."

It is a stalemate.

And then I write a story on my own and read it to Candis. A real, live story. Not homework—just me, expressing myself. Candis loves it. "Rate it," she demands, while she visibly holds her breath. I try to think about all of the positive aspects of the story. It is a solid piece; it's funny and it works. But I can't go there.

In a little voice, I say, "7 out of 10."

Candis looks at me with a determined and fierce look on her face. There is no beaming now, no compliments, no encouragement emanating from her. She is still, terrible, and quiet. The voice that comes from her is low and forceful and angry.

"When . . . are you . . . going . . . to stop . . . rating your writing . . . as a 7 out of 10?"

"When . . . are you . . . going . . . to stop . . . treating yourself . . . as a 7 out of 10?"

"When . . . are you . . . going . . . to stop . . . living your life . . . as a 7 out of 10?"

"When?" There is a dreaded pause between the thunder and the lightning. She slams her hand down on the table. "When?"

I sit there stunned. All my defenses are gone. Tears start pouring down my cheeks. And then I am sobbing. Big heavy sobs. My whole body is trembling. Snot runs down my face. I think inanely that I should have worn a raincoat. It is getting really wet in here.

I cannot fight it anymore. Candis loves my progress and my writing and me; she wants me to do the same. She doesn't see me as broken and hopeless. She sees the true me masked behind my deficits.

I learned the lessons from Candis, finally. It took me a long time. Life, hope, attitude, writing, sharing, dreaming . . . the list goes on and on. Mostly I have learned not to consider myself a 7 out of 10.

So now I have written this piece. It is time to read it and rate it. Hmmmm. It's not as good as I want it to be. Kind of awkward at points, but it does get its point across. Includes humor . . . expressive . . . honest . . . I give it . . . 8½ out of 10. At least!

Holly has published another story, which was also written as a therapy assignment, in the book *Chocolate for a Woman's Dreams*.

❧ ❧

**Embrace all aspects of healing.**
A skilled therapist will help you see that recovering from brain injury and learning to love your changed brain is not just about your body. It's important to pay attention to your mental, physical, emotional, social, and spiritual growth. Do not see yourself as a broken human being—a 7 out of 10. Recovering from stroke or brain injury is challenging, but you are still whole, strong, and capable of ongoing improvement in all areas of your life.

❧ "Quit beating yourself up."

STROKE THRIVER'S GROUP MEMBER

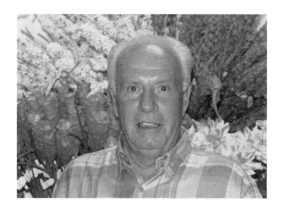

## Hope Empowers Stroke Survivors

*by* Herb

On the morning of the fifteenth of December 2006, I woke up
feeling tired. I couldn't decide whether to get up or be lazy and get
some more sleep. My eyes were open and my head was getting busy,
so I knew I had to get up. But once up, besides feeling tired, my
stomach felt squeamish and my bones felt old. I had washed up and
dressed, when all of a sudden I thought I was losing my eyesight.
I could see a big dull black spot. It quickly went away. This scared
me. I knew it wasn't a heart attack, but I didn't know what was
happening to me. I became very tired, but there was something
telling me to get out of the apartment. This was my inner voice
telling me to leave. I knew I had to be around people.

I could drive okay, but I felt really worn out. I never thought to
go to the hospital because I knew it wasn't a heart attack, but I never
thought of a stroke. I know now I should have called 911 instead of

driving my car. But I made it to the mall and stopped at Starbucks for a cup of coffee.

*I'm walking, carrying my coffee, when all of a sudden my right hand has no feeling in it. I drop the coffee, feeling embarrassed and thinking, "What is wrong with me? I have to get out of here." Now I'm terrified. I start walking, still no feeling in my hand. I feel very weak. My right leg starts to quiver; then it's shaking. My mind is racing. I come to the door that goes outside. My leg is shaking. Now my mind is saying, "What is going on?" I reach for the door. I can't reach it. I'm not there yet. I have to make it. I reach out again. It's there, but now I'm falling, falling.*

I have no idea how long I was out, but when I opened my eyes I was lying prone. I was very calm. I had my head on my arm. I couldn't talk. I was thinking, "Will I ever be able to talk again?" Someone was on her hands and knees, her face six inches from mine, her fingers in my hair telling me it was going to be okay. ("Maybe she knows something I don't," I thought.) I had no movement on my right side and very little movement on my left side. To me it was like being maybe one hundred feet in a tunnel surrounded by darkness, but being able to see light. Would I ever be able to walk, talk, or even move again?

When they put me on the stretcher, I couldn't feel any touching of my body. It was a two-block ride to the hospital. In the emergency room I remember a tube connected to my arm but no feeling.

*I'm starting to get scared again. The doctor is asking me all kinds of questions I can't answer. The doctor is looking nervous. He is pacing. It seems like a long time. The hospital tries to call my sister at home in California. As luck would have it my brother-in-law Rob is there. Rob is trying to contact my sister at work, who just happens to be out to lunch. There is only a three-hour window to administer the clot-buster medication. Rob reaches Pat, my sister, in time, and she gives the doctor permission to give me the drug. They give me the clot buster, and before they have half of it in me, I can feel my right arm and fingers moving, and then my left side moving.*

I could hear and feel myself crying. I could feel the wet tears on my face. My speech slowly came back. My tongue on the right was swollen, but it was a happy swollen. I was so happy to be able to feel it again.

After that evening, my sister and brother-in-law called me. I was still having a little trouble talking. I answered the phone from my hospital bed. My sister asked me how I was feeling. "Fine," I said, "just fine." My sister said, "FINE! FINE! What do you mean you're fine? Here we are, going ballistic, and you're fine?" What can I say? It is truly great to be alive.

After my stroke, my initial feeling was one of shame. I was struggling to get any words out. What will people think of me? I was still dealing with negative emotions following my early retirement from Northwest Airlines. Maybe it's just another bad thing in a line of bad things. But I also felt anger—why me? I don't deserve this.

I wondered, "What do I do? What can I do?" It was really hard for me to accept that the effects of the stroke were here to stay. I had always been athletic, and my body had let me down. Going into the hospital for rehab was really difficult. I had made it so big in my mind. I wasn't going to be able to conquer this overwhelming feeling of helplessness.

My first ray of hope came during visits from the stroke peer visitors while I was still in the hospital bed. Having these stroke survivor volunteers walk into my room made me realize I wasn't unique. There was hope, and I wanted some of what they had.

I started speech therapy at the hospital. My speech was slow and frustrating, but my speech therapist made me realize I wasn't dumb. She focused on my hobbies and interests. When I brought in some of my photographs, she made me realize that I did have other gifts. It was hard to recognize that I had other talents.

Occupational therapy helped me to recognize that lifting weights would strengthen my weak right arm and leg. I also got involved in a stroke Tai Chi exercise program at the hospital. It helps with relaxation, balance, and focusing my mind. I receive so much support from the people at Tai Chi.

**"My involvement in the other education and support programs helped me learn once again that I am not unique. There is help out there, but you have to ask for it."**

My involvement in the other education and support programs helped me learn once again that I am not unique. There is help out there, but you have to ask for it.

Now when I talk to people, I will ask them if they have emergency telephone numbers in their wallet. With these emergency numbers, someone can be contacted in order to give permission for any required procedure that could save your life. The bottom line is: What you don't have in your wallet could kill you.

With encouragement from my speech therapist, I bought a better camera and two great printers and launched my dream of creating photo greeting cards. I take pictures of flowers, landscapes, and people, then print and package them as cards and enlarged prints. I feel now that I have a lot of people who are cheering for me. I walk around with a glow inside me.

**Trust others.**

Herb reached out to others by engaging in rigorous therapy sessions and involving himself in group education, support sessions, and exercise classes with fellow survivors. The camaraderie and support of the people he met helped Herb deal with his negative emotions, including shame, anger, and helplessness.

The visit Herb received from the stroke peer visitors gave him confidence that he could recover. Stroke peer visitors are volunteers who are carefully selected and trained stroke survivors. Such first contacts with the stroke peer visitors often lay the groundwork for people to feel confident about seeking out support later. Group education, such as the StrokeWise classes, teach that stroke rehab is ongoing, and there is help along the way.

Peer visiting, classes, support groups, and aphasia conversation groups are offered to brain-injury survivors in many cities. Organizations such as the American Stroke Association, National Stroke Association, and the state department of health can be links to many different resources for stroke survivors.

> ᴥ "I feel badly for those who don't come out and seek education from groups. It's so important."
>
> STROKE THRIVER'S GROUP MEMBER

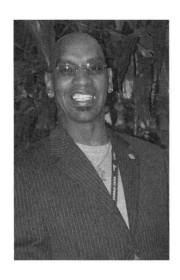

# Reaching Out to Others

*by* Stevie

In 1998, at age 35, I experienced a cerebral hemorrhage. A physically fit Army Reservist, I suddenly found that my left side was paralyzed. My speech, vision, and thinking process were all affected by the stroke, a cerebral hemorrhage that leaked blood into my brain. Stroke doesn't discriminate. It can happen to anyone at any age, regardless of race, gender, or health history. Accepting this fact is the first step to preventing stroke.

I was in five different health-care facilities over the next eight months. I found the physical and occupational therapy the most challenging. With my therapist Jill, I worked on isolating specific muscles and on high-level balance exercises. We walked outside together, up and down hills and on uneven surfaces and grass, to help with my ability to walk.

Though I did go through a period of feeling depressed right after the stroke, eventually I realized that my recovery was up to me.

**"There are some stumbling blocks on this journey, and you have to convert them to stepping-stones. It's about the experiences— going through them and embracing the good, the bad, the happy, and the sad parts of them."**

There are some stumbling blocks on this journey, and you have to convert them to stepping-stones. It's about the experiences—going through them and embracing the good, the bad, the happy, and the sad parts of them.

As I continued my recovery, I would visit the other patients at the facility I was staying in and talk to them. At the time, I didn't know that I was in training for the new life I would create for myself as a motivational speaker, lobbyist, stroke educator, group facilitator, and stroke peer mentor. As survivors, we speak the same language. And you learn from the people who've been over that bridge before.

I have taken my stroke experience and turned it into a positive experience. I didn't know my mission and purpose in life until after my stroke. Now I lobby locally every year for stroke research funding, and I've been to Washington, D.C. to lobby on a federal level. I'm a "Power to End Stroke Ambassador" and also on the Cultural Health Initiative Committee with the American Stroke Association. I give talks on the importance of stroke prevention to many audiences, especially within the African-American community, which has many risk factors for stroke.

Ultimately, I want people to learn how to pay attention to their lives so they get the most out of their journey. When you have something catastrophic happen, you think, "Just let me get through it." But I always tell people it's like driving: You see more at 55 miles per hour than at 90 miles per hour. It's the same with life. Embrace this moment. Think of all the good years you've had. You can have more, but you have to be open to what's ahead of you.

**Volunteer and advocate for others.**
Stevie shares his story with stroke survivors, their families, and the public, both to inspire and to help prevent stroke in others. Talking about your concerns builds relationships and can also result in systems, organizations, and policies changed for the better.

"Activism can help put anger and pain to work and shift our focus from blaming to helping. We can help ourselves at the same time we're helping others."
—Minnesota Brain Injury Association

  **"Helping others helps me."**

STROKE THRIVER'S GROUP MEMBER

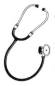

## TYPES OF STROKE

There are two types of strokes. A **hemorrhagic stroke** (bleeding into the brain) is caused by a broken blood vessel in or near your brain. This type of stroke may result from high blood pressure or a weakness in an artery wall (aneurysm) that causes the artery to balloon out and burst open.

An **ischemic stroke** is caused by a blockage in a blood vessel in the neck or brain. It is the most common type of stroke. It can be caused by high blood pressure, diabetes, problems with cholesterol, smoking, lack of physical activity, or excess weight. High blood pressure is a particularly significant but often overlooked risk factor for stroke. It often has no symptoms and is therefore called the "silent killer." Millions of people have high blood pressure and don't realize it. According to the American Medical Association, it affects 40 percent of African-American men and women over the age of 20.

Be sure you know the stroke signs and symptoms (see page 203). If the signs and symptoms last for a short period of time (a few minutes to less than 24 hours) it's called a **transient ischemic attack** (TIA). Having a TIA is a warning that you are at risk for a major stroke at any time. Seek medical attention right away at an emergency room.

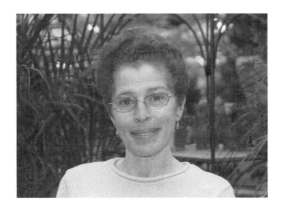

## One Piece of the Puzzle at a Time

*by* Debra

Having a stroke is a real trial, and everyone has to find their way of coping. I couldn't speak after my stroke. Reading was very difficult. Math was a nightmare. I was working out of a first grade workbook; this was the ultimate reality check.

Not being able to speak is a humbling experience. I was able to hear and understand what went on around me but was unable to respond. Frustration isn't a big enough word. Observing the frustration of family and friends who were worried about me wasn't easy. I wanted to let them know I was going to be all right.

Puzzles have always been an enjoyable pastime for me. Jigsaw, crossword, jumble, Sudoko—they were all enjoyable challenges. Aphasia is a puzzle I have to work my way around to communicate.

The hospital rehab program was a comfortable fit for me. The therapists and staff were so inviting. I felt really free to be myself.

Working hard to improve, but always finding humor in things that aren't easy, is therapy for me. Needing to test my comfort zone required me to talk to strangers.

My husband and I had just relocated from Wisconsin when I had my stroke, and we knew few people in Minnesota. Speaking and socializing were important pieces in my puzzle. Kurt works, and I did not want to talk to the cat all day. It was time to hit the streets. Every day was different, be it grocery shopping, driving to the mall, or walking to the dry cleaners. One thing was the same: I had to have small conversations with at least two people. This was a confidence builder. Once in a while I met up with a sourpuss, but a negative outcome is better than no outcome at all. Since we were new to the area, we'd take tours on the weekend. Group tours were most challenging because I'd have to ask a question in front of a group of people.

**"Being ready to take a chance and to be uncomfortable for a while helped me through some rough times."**

Being ready to take a chance and to be uncomfortable for a while helped me through some rough times. It is easier now for me to have casual conversations. However, two years have passed, and when I'm tired, ill, or the noise level is uncomfortable for me, I remind myself, "one piece of the puzzle at a time."

**Challenge yourself to grow through the frustrating times.**
Frustration is a sign you are challenging yourself to improve.
Even though she found it uncomfortable at times, Debra's
willingness to move out of her comfort zone enhanced her
communication progress. You can benefit by setting daily
goals for yourself, as Debra did for herself. Games, puzzles,
conversations, and group interaction all make for good rehab
therapy, with you as your own best therapist.

❧ "It is so affirming to hear of others' similar frustrations.
Groups for stroke survivors are great. I feel blessed
to be able to both give and receive support."

STROKE THRIVER'S GROUP MEMBER

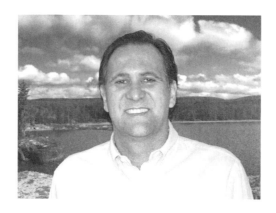

# How It Feels to Eat and Drink Again

*by* Vido

At age 45, I was an active person and owner of a coffee-distribution company and a plantation in Brazil. I had two strokes. They left me with compromised speech and the inability to swallow foods and liquids. I had to have a tube in my stomach to ensure adequate nutrition and hydration.

I regained consciousness several days after my stroke. My wife said to me, "You are fortunate, only 10 percent of people live after that kind of stroke."

My stroke resulted in **dysphagia** (difficulty swallowing). At first liquids and foods would not go down. Yes, I could swallow, but not fast enough to prevent food and liquid from going into my lungs. I didn't have the strength to cough and was not aware that food was going into my airway.

I practiced tongue and throat exercises rigorously, hoping I could swallow. I went home and exercised diligently. With therapy,

I discovered I could swallow small amounts of food. My liquids were thickened, so they did not go into my lungs. In out-patient therapy with a speech-language pathologist, I had my first thin liquid via a teaspoon. I was so excited. I knew it wouldn't be long before I could drink from a cup. Only seven weeks after my stroke, I can enjoy a cup of cappuccino one sip at a time. My stomach tube has been removed, and I can eat and drink independently. Now, when food and liquids come close to my airway, I have a strong cough.

Because of swallowing therapy, I can now swallow chips with salsa, peanuts, dried fruit, and, best of all, I can drink water and coffee. All textures are great gifts.

My wife is not a nurse and has not had the training of a nurse, but she loves me and is there walking beside me. She makes all the difference. I don't know where I'd be if it wasn't for her. I love her so much.

"Because of swallowing therapy, I can swallow chips with salsa, peanuts, dried fruit, and, best of all, I can drink water and coffee. All textures are great gifts."

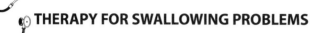

## THERAPY FOR SWALLOWING PROBLEMS

Aspirating food and liquids into the lungs can cause serious problems, including lung infections and pneumonia. Right after his stroke, Vido was put on a feeding tube to keep him strong and healthy while he was in therapy. This saved Vido's life, since his swallow wasn't working and he was unable to cough productively. In therapy Vido practiced "tongue aerobic" exercises. He was taught to swallow hard, as if there were a ping-pong ball in his throat and he needed to get it down. He learned swallowing strategies to get his throat going again. Speech-language pathologists recommend the following to help with swallowing:

- Eat slowly and chew food thoroughly.

- Eat in an upright position.

- Preparing food in a certain way, or avoiding certain foods may help. For example, you may have to avoid hot or cold foods or drinks.

- If you cannot swallow liquids properly, you may need to add special thickeners to your drinks.

- Use any swallowing techniques you have been taught by a speech-language pathologist to fit your particular swallowing problem.

- Take any medicine prescribed for your problem as directed. If the medicines are not working or are causing side effects, let your healthcare provider know.

- If you have new or different symptoms, tell your healthcare provider right away.

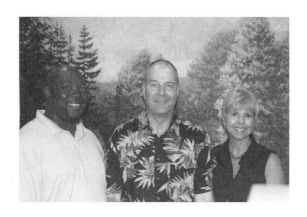

# A Team Effort

*by* John F., Linda, and Deondray

John shares his experience:

I was sleeping. I wasn't even aware of what was going on. My wife, Linda, knew something was wrong, but didn't know what was happening to me. That was almost five years ago. The stroke put me in bed for three months. I couldn't communicate. I couldn't move my arms or walk. Now I'm able to rise up from my wheelchair, communicate with simple words, gestures, and facial expressions, walk short distances, and move my right side. I understand speech and I have a great sense of humor. Before my stroke, I was a salesman for the Minnesota Wild Hockey Association, and I loved to talk. Communication now is steady—much better than at the beginning. Now I can watch a movie and tell what I saw in the movie. I can tell you what I want to eat and what I don't want to eat, and I can hold a conversation with my old employees.

My children tickle my funny bone. I have a great group of kids. They have patience with my disabilities.

Deondray is a Certified Nursing Assistant and home health aide. He has worked with John as his carepartner for the past four years. John communicates with gestures, facial expressions, smiles, laughter, and a limited vocabulary. John, his wife Linda, and Deondray work as a team. Linda believes Deondray has developed a magical relationship with her husband—one that is filled with respect, love, and commitment.

Deondray says he looks at life differently after working with John. He shares some lessons he's learned from his friend:

- Love your family, because you never know what could happen to change that person.

- Value life, because you never know. Many people think, "I can put that off until tomorrow." Tomorrow may be different than you've planned.

- Have patience and understanding.

- Keep open communication in your family, because if everyone is aware of what is going on, then unexpected situations can be handled better.

- It is important to have a loving family who understands, no matter what.

- There is still a life after a stroke—you just have to work harder.

Linda is John's wife of 38 years. The couple has two children. She writes about her husband's stroke:

As we approach the five-year mark since John's stroke, I'm still amazed that if I close my eyes I can relive the entire experience, detail by detail, all over again, as if it only just happened. When life changes so dramatically, sometimes the only way to make sense of it is to replay it over and over. I used to do that quite a lot at first. Not so much anymore.

What I've learned is that recovery and healing are not easily measured and are not the same for everyone. John suffered a severe stroke, the result of a blood clot dislodged by a condition called atrial fibrillation (a kind of irregular heartbeat). He was in a deep coma, fighting for his life, for almost an entire week. His team of doctors told our two children and me that the damage to his brain was so extensive that he had a poor chance of recovery— and if he did live, we should plan to place him in a nursing home for the rest of his days. They were wrong. After three weeks in an intensive care unit, four months at a rehab hospital, and six months at a transitional rehabilitation center, we brought John home.

**"Our plans and dreams have all changed now. But they didn't die. We are closer than ever and love each other more now. We are thankful to be together."**

Although the stroke left John with right-side paralysis and expressive aphasia, he's made amazing progress. He walks, with help, and his speech continues to improve to this day. The stroke also left him with an increased zest for life and a wonderful sense of humor. I tease him that he is funnier now than he ever was. And being married for 38 years, we pretty much know what the other one is thinking most of the time anyway, so our communication is good.

Do I miss the old John? You bet I do. We were truly partners who shared everything in our marriage, from paying the bills to household chores. I miss being able to talk over financial issues, decisions about our kids, or challenges in my job. The burden is heavy when you carry it alone. But I look back on our long marriage and know that many times over those years, John carried more than his share of the same burden. It's what a promise is all about. He's still a good listener, a caring and sensitive man, and even if he can't solve a problem, knowing I still have him to talk to is enough. Our plans and dreams have all changed now. But they didn't die. We are closer than ever and love each other more now. We are thankful to be together. Life is certainly different than we ever imagined. But at the end of every day, we can still kiss each other good night and hold hands as we fall asleep. And who knows. Some day soon, he may take me out dancing one more time.

❧ ❧

**Choose positive words to describe your new life.**
The words we use are powerful and affect how we see ourselves. "Stroke survivor" reinforces the strength and fortitude it takes to live with the challenges of stroke. The word "victim" suggests weakness. A survivor, or a "thriver," knows the strength of character required each day and strives to reach each milestone on the climb to the mountain peak. John, Linda, and Deondray use the words "carepartner" instead of "caregiver" or "caretaker." The term "carepartner" preserves the dignity of the stroke survivor and recognizes how much they still have to give others.

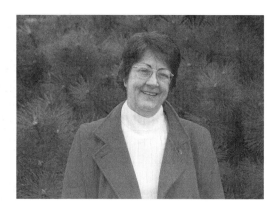

# Not That Bad

*by* Maxine

After my stroke in August, 2005, I was told that I had aphasia and disability with my right hand and leg. Aphasia? Aphasia affects reading, writing, speaking, listening, numbers, and memory, among other things. Stubbornly, I thought, I can't be "that bad." I didn't feel "that bad."

After my initial time in the hospital, I spent three weeks in rehab. I worked hard to prove I was not "that bad." I began to hear of my improvement from family, friends, and counselors.

Little victories came from figuring out the telephone. Bigger victories came from writing my name and using my right hand. My aphasia had me stumped: "peek-a-boo" became "pook-a-bee"; "yes" became "no"; "23" became "32." Big words got jumbled. Numbers were a challenge. There was a lot of "Sorry, you have the wrong number."

My old singing voice is a thing of the past. I can sing to myself, but I can't carry a tune and keep up with the song lyrics. Certain words will come up wrong.

A sense of humor is necessary. We laughed a lot that first year. And thanks to my rehabilitation at the hospital and patience, understanding, and a sense of humor from my family and friends, I can finally say, "I'm not that bad."

Life has slowed down a little, but I am still active. I can drive, I can cook (carefully), clean house, and all those fun things. I love gardening, and I volunteer my time. I have my family and friends. God just made me change lanes, and appreciate what I have. It gets better and better. Keep on plugging along. Maybe I'll even try a little speech refresher course to enhance my speech abilities.

❧ ☙

### Consider a different kind of work.

Maxine spent 20 years working for a county Adult Probation Office. After her stroke, she began working in a bakery. It's very different from any kind of work she'd done before, but it provides her with structure during her week and a place where she can socialize. She also volunteers at StrokeWise classes for stroke survivors, and shows compassion and understanding for class participants who struggle to find their words. If you are unable to continue doing the work you did before your stroke, consider another type of job that might offer you structure, social contacts, and a place to practice your communication skills.

❧ **"Returning to work is a double-edged sword. It's good to be with people and enjoy the job, but tasks can be so challenging."**
STROKE THRIVER'S GROUP MEMBER

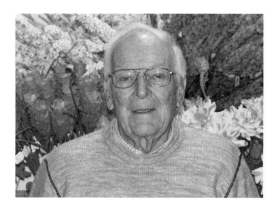

# Tips for Stroke Thrivers and Their Families

*by* John W.

John is a stroke survivor, and he has worked hard in recovery from aphasia. He has volunteered once a week as a stroke peer visitor at the hospital for almost six years. John feels strongly that we can all send important messages to new stroke survivors with our words and our attitude. Here he offers us his tips.

Don't get discouraged—this condition will likely improve. Recovery is different for each stroke survivor. Every person is different and every stroke is different. After volunteering as a stroke peer visitor, I've learned the most important thing is to be positive.

Don't talk about the person and their stroke within their hearing: "This could have killed him. I don't think she's gonna make it." Rather, talk about your personal feelings outside the room, and always be upbeat with the survivor. Find something they did right so you can congratulate them for achieving. I was so taken by the fact that I couldn't talk, I didn't even notice that the stroke had affected my arm and leg. I was thunderstruck. I couldn't get my feelings and ideas across. They wouldn't let me up, so I couldn't do anything for myself. *Awful.*

Nothing has ever hit me as hard as the first days of my stroke. Am I going to live? There is a lot of fear, and it could be several months before you really understand what deficits develop because of the stroke. But most people get much better than they are in the first few days.

Most thoughts come out in words. It's frustrating to think about something that you can't speak. The first few days are very frustrating to a stroke survivor who has aphasia.

For the visitor: Talk to the individual with aphasia as if he understands you. He probably does, even though he can't talk himself.

Show a lot of hope, because that's all he has at this point. Get him going in a hopeful direction.

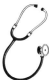

## THE BRAIN AND LANGUAGE

Various areas of your brain contribute to your ability to understand and use language. A stroke may damage only those areas related to reproducing words, while leaving the areas that allow you to understand language intact and fully functional. In such a case, you would not be able to talk, but you would be able to comprehend what was said to you.

For this reason, it is advisable to discuss a survivor's prognosis in a separate room. Make sure to encourage survivors and celebrate their progress. Making a sound after being silent for a day is huge progress. Saying a word is an even bigger achievement.

While a survivor is still in the hospital, families should be encouraged to spend time with the patient. They can provide moral support that is crucial during the first days after stroke. Families should seek information from doctors in order to fully understand the extent of injury to the brain. Then they can be better prepared to support the patient's recovery.

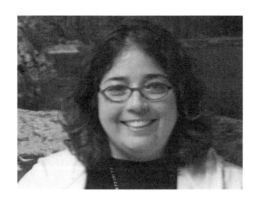

# Word Lists

*by* Claudia

Claudia was asked to write a list of random words that described her life for a therapeutic writing assignment. Then she was told to use those words in a story. Her word list and story are below.

discovery

new life

memory issues

keeping track of time and schedule

meeting new people

finding new hobbies

financial concerns

grief and loss, letting go of old life

getting to know parents

inability to drive anymore

dependency on others

cleaning out closet

I am very worried about several issues going on in my life at this time. At the forefront is my inability to work in the field I went to school for, which in turn has created financial concerns. I am no longer able to work as a social worker because I am unable to drive anymore, and keeping track of time and schedules, writing court reports, etc., became difficult as a result of memory issues and word retrieval. I am going through grief and loss at letting go of my old life. I am in a discovery period, learning to become dependent on others, meeting new people, finding new hobbies, and tackling a large dilemma of cleaning out a closet that has become bloated with clothes I no longer use. I need to focus on a new life. Despite all these new challenges, a positive thing has occurred: I have gotten to know my parents better and the love they have for me.

My hopes and dreams for my future are to continue learning and experiencing what my new life has to offer—e.g., helping my father create a website for the publications he completed while a professor at the University of Minnesota. I also look forward to discovering the new me and the woman I can become.

My name is Claudia. I was born in Iowa City on April 4, 1966, along with my twin sister. My family moved to the state of Minnesota prior to my attending kindergarten. My family is originally from Chile, and Spanish was the first language I learned to speak.

I graduated from university with a double major in psychology and photography. I worked for several years after this in student loans, then decided that I wanted a different direction for my life and attended graduate school at the Alfred Adler School. Then I began my career in adult mental health.

In 2003 I was diagnosed with multiple sclerosis. My hope for the future is to continue to be a productive individual and enjoy my life experiences.

A year and a half later, I'm doing better. Mentally I'm better. Medically it's challenging, as I continue to lose my eyesight. It's hard to adjust to a new lifestyle of being dependent on people, yet it's shown me how blessed I am to know how much people love me. Even though it has been a challenge, it has been good, too, because I don't take things for granted. At times I feel isolated, because I am no longer able to drive, and my friends work. I meet with them when I can, and I appreciate what I do get.

I have gotten organized. I write my thoughts down in a journal and write word lists. If I use the wrong word, I make a joke. I take a letter of the alphabet, write it down, and think of words that begin with that letter. My niece is eight years old and very articulate. She takes the words that I write and makes up a silly story that makes me laugh. It's a fun way to spend time together: She learns words, and I get to see her develop as a little human being with a wonderful sense of humor.

❧ ☙

### Make a word list to practice writing.

A functional therapeutic strategy you can try is to list 10 to 20 words randomly and use them in a story. The outcome is often a heartfelt story like Claudia's, which enhances your memory and use of vocabulary. It also helps with thought organization and the sequencing of ideas, both challenges with Claudia's Multiple Sclerosis, very similar to aphasia. You might be surprised at how a list of random words can flow into a rich personal story that can become a keepsake for you and your family members.

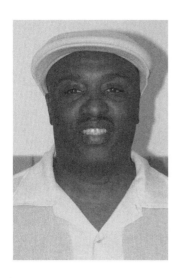

# Give Your Brain a Break

*by* Danny

When I got home from the hospital after my first stroke, I wanted to get on with my life. I was involved in therapy, and I thought I could do it on my own at home. I had a second small stroke in April 2008, and suddenly I discovered I needed to learn more about stroke and how I could speed up my recovery. I enrolled in a StrokeWise class.

I've learned what to eat and what not to eat in order to stay strong and decrease my risk of stroke. I know when to rest and when to take it slow to reserve my energy. I discovered that thinking makes me tired. I learned about the brain, and I'm reminded that I'm to "Kiss my brain." If I give my brain a "brain break," it will work much better. Brain breaks are those necessary pauses for rest that refuel, rejuvenate, and refresh my brain so it works better.

**"If I give my brain a 'brain break,' it will work much better. Brain breaks are those necessary pauses for rest that refuel, rejuvenate, and refresh my brain so it works better."**

I applied everything I learned in stroke rehab therapy to my life. There are many simple ways to make life productive after a stroke. Do two or three of the strategies that work for you. For example, when I first had my stroke I had double vision and couldn't walk or talk. Now when I'm walking I can't just look straight ahead or I miss things. I turn to the left or turn to the right but don't look down or I'll lose my balance.

I was home, my wife worked. I wanted to help. In occupational therapy I learned how to screw tops on and off and to pick up small objects. I practiced picking up peanuts as therapy. It helped with hand coordination to move the peanuts from hand to hand. I learned to open Ramen noodles. Also, I swept and mopped daily, which helped with arm strength and coordination. I played basketball; the dribbling and shooting helped my eye/hand coordination. Washing dishes helped with hand skills. I cleaned sinks and dusted. I could feel different textures—rough/smooth, hot/cold. Sometimes I couldn't feel hot and cold, because my brain didn't get the signal. When washing clothes, I carried laundry up and down the steps to help with balance.

I use a tape recorder to listen, recall, and remember details. If too much information comes at me too quickly I may lose an important idea. I advise anyone to participate in stroke classes, because they help you deal with your life. The love and care feels great. You try harder. I want to be a thriver, not a quitter. Others can help me in my quest for information, which helps me heal faster.

**Save your energy and spend it wisely.**
Every stroke is different, but stroke survivors often have one thing in common: fatigue. It's that sleepiness or overwhelming feeling of exhaustion that just won't go away.

We all have a limited amount of energy in our energy bank. These energy reserves may be even more limited after a brain injury, so it's important to spend them wisely. Save enough energy to do the things you enjoy, such as hobbies or lunch with a friend.

Don't become discouraged by fixating on what your life was like before your stroke. Energy comes from enthusiasm and joy. Exercise your enthusiasm by rewarding yourself every day for your successes. Then, make better use of the energy you *do* have by practicing energy strategies like those listed below:

- Spend time with people who make you feel good.

- Make sure you are comfortable and free of pain and distractions at night so you can sleep better.

- Take a nap during the day, if it gives you more energy and doesn't leave you feeling worse.

- Spread heavy and light tasks throughout the day and the week.

- Plan only one heavy or high-energy task per day at the most.

- Remember, "heavy" tasks may now include shopping, vacuuming, yard work, and laundry.

- Write down tasks, and decide which are the most important.

- Schedule rest breaks into your day.

- Steer clear of activities you can't stop if you tire out (for example, cleaning out the garage).

- Ask for help if you need it.

- Avoid rushing and unneeded tasks.

- Sit to work whenever possible.

- Use stress management techniques. (See page 152.)

- Keep items used often within easy reach.

- Try exercising for just 10 minutes at a time. Do this two or three times each day.

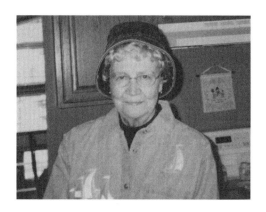

# Storms of Life

*by* Nancy

Nancy writes about her mother, Jeanne. After her stroke, Jeanne faced her therapy challenges with determination, courage, and grace. She never gave up.

My mother was very afraid of storms, high winds, and tornadoes. As a kid, I remember going down into the basement when the storms were severe. Even as an adult, whenever I was at her house and the weather was bad, we would go down into the basement, with the radio and the dog and wait for the weather to improve. However, when storms came up in my mom's personal life, she did not show any fear.

Mom's first personal storm was in 1991, when she was diagnosed with breast cancer. Her next personal storm happened on April 15, 2002, when my mom suffered a stroke. She was lucky enough to be at her job at a medical clinic when the symptoms started. She later said that as she was putting on her lipstick at home, she felt a little funny, and driving to work she felt strange. When she was at the clinic, she spilled her coffee, felt a little dizzy, and found her speech didn't make any sense. Her co-worker knew that something was not right and ran to get the doctor. The doctor that the co-worker ran back to get happened to be Mom's doctor. He was the one that told her what was going on. They called 911, took her to the Emergency Room, and then called me.

At the hospital, the doctor examined Mom and verified that she was having a stroke. She explained to us about this new drug, tPA, which, if taken within three hours of symptoms, might reverse all or some of the effects of the stroke. There was also a risk of internal bleeding, if I am recalling this correctly.

My brother and I did not know what to do. I remember thinking, "Where is Debbie [my sister, the nurse]?" We told the doctor to go ahead with the clot-buster medication, and then Debbie walked in. Thank God! She had heard of the drug and said to go ahead and give it to her. We would not know until the next day if it worked. That day was one of the worst days of our lives. My mom knew what was going on and was crying. She did not want to be like this. Her right side was affected—her face, arm, and leg. She kept repeating the same words. They were: *home*, *dog*, and *car*. I knew what she meant. Her car was at her job, she wanted it back home. She wanted someone to go take care of her dog. She also kept saying she was sorry. This broke my heart. She was the one having a stroke, and she was apologizing to us. It was terrible to see her like that. The entire family came: her brother and sister and their spouses. We prayed all day and took turns going into her room to see her. It was a long, long day. Finally, at around 8:00 p.m., I went home to do what she wanted, get the car and take care of the dog. We all went home that night and prayed for Mom and for the tPA to work.

Well, our prayers were answered. The drug worked. When Johnny, my brother, and I walked into her room the next morning, Mom was sitting up in bed smiling. She said, "Hi," and was eating breakfast with her right hand (her affected side). She was doing great, except for her speech. She had aphasia. Her speech was the only thing that had not been totally reversed. The doctor came in and was amazed at Mom's progress. She examined Mom and explained what was happening with her speech. She told us what aphasia was and informed Mom that she would have speech therapy. The first question Mom asked the doctor was, "Can I go back to work?" and the doctor said, "Yes, you will be going back to work."

I believe this one sentence from the doctor gave Mom the incentive, strength, and hope to get through what was ahead. I do not believe in coincidences. We all saw God working that day of her stroke. After the hospital, Mom went to a rehabilitation clinic. This was not pleasant for Mom, as she wanted to be in her own home and be with her dog, Sandi. But she applied herself to whatever they wanted her to do. She had speech, occupational, and physical therapy.

My mom was the strongest woman I know. Not once did she complain about what happened to her—she only said she wanted to go home. My mom went home on April 24, 2002. It was a great day for our entire family. Mom was thrilled to be in her own home with her dog.

We kept a journal for about a month starting from the day she came home. This is why I can remember some of the details. Mom had occupational therapy for about a week, and then she was fine to be on her own. She also received speech therapy at home and eventually as an out-patient. Again we saw the handprints of God, as her speech therapist was an amazing and wonderful person.

Mom had homework from her speech therapist and would sometimes get frustrated that she could not understand all of it. I would look at her homework, and it was hard for me.

She worked very hard on her speech with her therapist and throughout this entire time Mom did not complain. She was always positive about what was going on with her. Her faith was so strong and grew stronger every day.

However, before she could go back to work, she was hit by another storm. She was diagnosed with uterine cancer. She was not scheduled for surgery until the third week in August, so Mom went back to work. She had done it. She had accomplished her goal. She only worked a week and a half and then went in for surgery.

I would like to point out a few things regarding her stroke. First, her life was saved because she was at the hospital within the three-hour window for the clot-busting medication. This is very important. You only have three hours after the stroke occurs to get this drug, and she did. The second thing was, her doctor gave her hope and a goal to push for. The third thing was the speech therapist who inspired and befriended my mom. She knew what Mom wanted and gave her hard assignments to help her do this.

When Mom had the surgery, she was diagnosed with Stage 4 uterine cancer. This cancer could not be cured, only slowed down. For the next two years, Mom went through chemotherapy to maintain her life. Always a fighter! Unfortunately, her storms were not done yet. The doctor diagnosed Mom with Parkinson's disease the last six weeks of her life. Three days after Thanksgiving, on November 29, 2004, Mom passed away at her home surrounded by her loving family and beloved dog, Sandi.

Through all the storms in her life—cancer, stroke, cancer, and Parkinson's disease—she never felt sorry for herself or asked "Why me?" She fought every storm that came her way. I said it before and I will say it again: She is the strongest woman I have ever known, and I am proud to call her my mother. Her courage, strength, and faith are a true inspiration to me. Hopefully her story will help others with the storms in their lives.

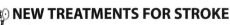

## NEW TREATMENTS FOR STROKE

How a stroke is treated in the hospital depends on when the stroke started, what the symptoms are, the capabilities of the hospital, and a number of other factors. Some stroke centers will have neurointerventional radiology services able to provide the treatments described here.  There are three main procedures doctors might use, but an angiogram must be done first.

An angiogram involves threading a tiny tube from a small opening in the artery at the top of the thigh and up through the arteries to the location of the blockage. Contrast dye and x-ray identify where the blockage is. The doctor will then decide which treatment option would be the best to use for different areas and types of blockage. Sometimes all three treatments are used in the same patient. Patients are screened very closely by the doctor to make sure they would be a good candidate for any of these procedures.

There are three options for treatment of a stroke while it is happening:

- injection of alteplase (tPA) into the artery

- use of a device called the Merci Retriever

- use of a device called the Penumbra System.

In all three treatments, a tube is inserted next to the blockage in the artery near or in the brain. Alteplase, more commonly referred to as tPA, is a strong, clot-busting medication. It can be injected into the clot to break it up or dissolve it. Interarterial tPA must be given within six hours of the onset of stroke symptoms to avoid some complications. tPA medication given through a vein must be given within three hours. The biggest risk with tPA is bleeding in the brain. This risk can increase the longer oxygen is blocked from getting to parts of the brain. The possibility for damage to brain tissue increases after six hours.

The Merci Retriever looks like a corkscrew. It, too, is used inside the blood vessels. The tiny corkscrew device is inserted into the clot, and the doctor then attempts to pull the clot out. This device can be used within eight hours of the onset of stroke symptoms.

The Penumbra System is also used inside the blood vessels. It uses a vacuum suction to remove or pull the blockage out. It should also be used within eight hours of the onset of stroke symptom.

Generally, these procedures are used when the blocked blood vessel is large. It is difficult to use the retrieval and vacuum devices in the tiny arteries in the brain. Usually, if it is a large blood vessel, the symptoms are very noticeable. Risks of the above procedures include bleeding into the brain and damage to a blood vessel. The risks can increase as time passes. Patients are watched very closely throughout the procedure by the doctor, nurses, and technicians.

Despite the risks, in some cases the outcome is very good with these new techniques, with stroke deficits decreasing dramatically from the original symptoms. New treatments for stroke are continuing to develop rapidly as research moves forward. If interested, you may call your local hospital to ask if they provide these neurointerventional treatments.

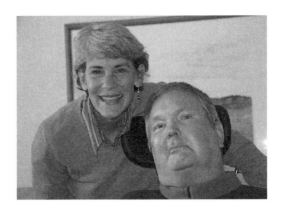

# Finding Faith

*by* Cliff

Hello, my name is Cliff. I'm 57 years old and a nonverbal quadriplegic, living in a group home. I am married to a wonderful, caring wife of almost 29 years, and have four great children, ranging in age from 27 to 17. I also am a former high school teacher and coach of basketball and softball, and have enjoyed writing screenplays, a website, and, more recently, newsletter articles. I have used a head-control computer, which is put on the bridge of my glasses. When the infrared device is connected with a camera, it activates the mouse and I am able to write.

Unfortunately, because of my physical situation, I have to live away from my family. You see, in June of 1992, I suffered a brainstem stroke. It left me paralyzed from the neck down and cost me the ability to speak. Apparently, it rates number one as the worst kind of stroke. Most people experiencing this stroke die. That made me a bit of a novelty to many of the doctors, since I lived.

One of the main things I've learned is that money and fame are empty attempts at finding meaning to your life. I had heard that said before suffering this stroke, but I only believed it on an intellectual level. On a gut level, I believed these things were important to personal happiness. My realization came in being at the doorstep of death. I can honestly say that when you look death in the eyes, the size of your checkbook or your status in society becomes irrelevant.

The other extremely important thing I've learned is to know the one thing we can control, and practice it in our lives as well. A few months before I had the stroke, I read the book *Man's Search For Meaning* by the German psychiatrist Viktor Frankl. It was about his survival in a Nazi concentration camp. He believed that most things in life happen outside our control, and accepting that is crucial to avoid being saddled with anxiety and hopelessness. The irony is the simplicity of tapping into the strength we can have by utilizing the one thing we can control, and that is our attitude. We often try to control what we can't and ignore what we can. He accepted the reality that his life was in the hands of the Nazis, but they could only control his spirit if he surrendered it. That was the control that got his focus, and not the presence of the Nazis.

This philosophy is what I've tried to live by during the last almost fifteen years of my life. Throughout this adventure, people have been interested in my different point of view. I remember a friend saying, "Your stroke has been so unusual that it is like you visited another planet." One can only imagine the enormous amount of experiences I have had, living first at hospitals and rehab centers, then at nursing homes, and now at a group home. Through no desire on my part, the overriding activity of my days is thinking—about

15 to 17 hours out of every 24. It isn't that I want to, but I can do nothing to stop it. It's funny to me now, that when I taught, I'd talk to students about thinking more. Now being an airhead for a day is a matter of envy.

I remember a time when diversions to ease the mind, like touch football or shooting a basketball, were common. At this point in my life, there's no escape. One might argue whether this time I have been given is a blessing or a curse. Over time I have decided to consider it a gift and put it to good use, and pray. I certainly had spent time in prayer before my stroke, but not several hours a day. God and I have become great friends.

Physically, I have reflected on the absurdity of my situation. I couldn't possibly do justice to describing the utter insanity of the type of problems that sometimes haunt me every day. Think of the simple way you might take care of a minor itch on your forehead or an insignificant cramp in your hamstring and imagine what it might be like not to be able to do anything about it. If you can do this, you can get some insight into a typical day for me. During the summer months in Minnesota, dealing with insects makes me feel absolutely defenseless. I feel powerless to do anything. A mosquito will land on my arm. I watch it suck blood from me, like it was a vampire, and then it flies away. I have no idea of its final destination. As far as I know, it is excitedly out recruiting other mosquitoes. Another huge thing is not being able to be in bed with my wife, or being able to play with our kids. Not doing this is not only strange, but very hard.

Eating is another issue that is always a challenge. I have gone from receiving my daily sustenance from a feeding tube (where I lost 50 pounds—not a method of losing weight I'd recommend), to eating nursing home food, to eating the much more palatable food of a group home, with a myriad of feeding and drinking techniques to help lessen the possibility of choking. I am thankful I can eat now. I never knew I could be so grateful for something so simple.

My years in nursing homes would be impossible to explain. Suffice it to say, my days were filled with huge miscommunications with all staff. On a regular basis, I would get blamed for things I couldn't possibly have done (DUH! Since I'm a quadriplegic!). I do admit to being ungrateful, and even rude at times, because of the total frustration of the details of my life. But one day in 1998, I began having a sense of peace and calm that I couldn't describe. It was different than anything I'd ever experienced. Situations occurred where I knew I just needed to forgive. Justice will come later. In spite of all the indignities suffered, I was overwhelmed with a sense of forgiveness and keeping things light. Every day revealed a more relaxed attitude from me, and fewer outbursts. I increasingly utilized my faith in God to witness miracles happen.

I began having changing thoughts. I loved seeing my family. I began recalling little crazy things we used to do. I spent long hours thinking about how I could have been a much better husband, father, and friend. At times I was more focused on myself, rather than focusing on others. The tragedy was that it took being near death to realize their importance. Personally, I was mad at myself for wasting time with meaningless pursuits that so easily could seduce me into believing they were important.

In hindsight, I'll always be grateful to some very special people for generously getting me a computer and, more recently, a "talker." Having movement in my head gave me the ability to use them. This fact is very important because, for a few hours each day, I have had an outlet for much of what I feel. Besides writing screenplays, having a website, and newsletter articles, I also can write and receive e-mails from my family and friends. This is especially helpful, since, after the onset of my stroke, I can finally focus more on the important relationships in my life. Getting my mind off of myself is huge. Most recently, I have needed to take a break from the use of my computer and "talker," mainly because of long-standing fatigue, depression, and medical complications from the stroke.

"Before the stroke, I thought happiness was found in personal achievement. Now, I live with an inner peace that can't be explained because it's beyond understanding."

Before the stroke, I thought happiness was found in personal achievement. Now, I live with an inner peace that can't be explained because it's beyond understanding. My earthly happiness comes from something very simple. I love being with my wife and our kids. I like seeing the glow on their faces. I also love hearing what they have to say. I know they'll make me laugh. In the early years of the stroke, I became aware that very little makes me afraid. Now, there's even less. I especially don't find death scary. I only find being without God scary. All in all, I'm not going to quit. I'll always pray, and never give up.

**You *can* control your attitude.**

No matter how challenging your life is, you have the power to choose to look at it in a positive way. Cliff draws strength from the love of his wife and children and his faith in God. He has bad days, of course, but he chooses to keep reminding himself of the things he has to be grateful for.

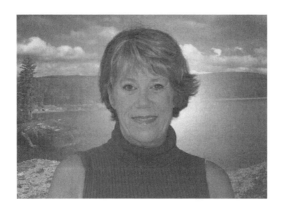

## Slow but Steady

*by* Janet

I LOVE TO TALK!

As a youngster in school the teachers often said, "Janet, keep quiet and listen." I always sat in the back of the classroom so I could talk during class. When the report card came out, it always indicated how much I talked, and my mom would ask, "Janet, why do you talk so much in school?" As an adult, I was a leader in conversations. My way with words could always get people to listen.

Six months ago I had a stroke and was unable to talk; it was horrible. The words were all messed up. I did not realize I was calling everyone by my sister's name, "Carol." Everyone was "she" when I meant "he." Everything I was saying came out "buttons."

So I had to start slow, and I had to talk slow, which was not me. I always did everything fast. When I talked too fast, my words got all messed up and mumbled. I used to work fast, talk fast, type fast, and eat fast. Everything was done fast. That was me, my personality.

Now that six months have passed since my stroke, I have learned to slow down a bit. It has been very hard for me to remember the new way of life—slow motion.

**"I had to start slow, and I had to talk slow, which was not me. I always did everything fast."**

I have improved so much because of my determination to get back to my old self. Even now, I find it hard to slow down. I have learned that everything does not have to be done quickly. I can take my time doing things that I love to do, and it doesn't have to be hurried. My lifestyle has changed for me. Smell the roses.

❧ ❧

**Recovery is not a race.**
The rate of recovery and the end results will be different for everyone with a brain injury. The location and size of the brain injury will determine many of your challenges. But, like Janet, your determination will greatly affect your recovery. Rehab is hard work. Give yourself the time you need to accomplish the goals you set for yourself. As Janet discovered, it is often better to pay attention to each moment, instead of running as fast as you can.

❧ "Measure success in small steps."
STROKE THRIVER'S GROUP MEMBER

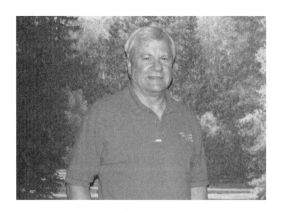

## Finding My Balance

*by* Dave

It started as just an ordinary day, September 7, 2005. I was getting ready for work. The bathroom sink was clogged up, so I used a strong drain cleaner and had gotten some on my hands. It made my hands kind of tingle, but I didn't think too much of it.

At about 10:30 that morning I started to feel different at work. My walking seemed strange, and I had to really concentrate when someone talked to me. As the day went on, I mentioned to fellow co-workers that I didn't feel right. Finally, at about 4:30 p.m., I decided to go home. I got in my van to drive home in busy traffic. That drive home was a real task. I lay down for a while, but that didn't seem to help. We ate dinner and I tried to watch TV. We were leaving on a trip the next day, and my wife was getting ready for that. She kept checking on me but kept asking questions relating to heart attacks, for which I had no symptoms. Later, she called poison control regarding the chemical I used. They suggested we call for medical help, as the chemical should not produce those symptoms.

My wife's friend called, and when she told her about me, her friend's daughter, who is a nurse, said, "Go to the hospital."

The next days were very fuzzy. I know they ran a lot of tests and an MRI. I had lost feeling on my left side, both the arm and leg, and also felt confused. I was unable to stand alone or walk, and had trouble gathering my thoughts.

I do remember getting a visit from a stroke survivor named John. I remember thinking that I couldn't tell he'd had a stroke, so there was hope for me.

After a few more days, I was transferred to another hospital for acute rehab therapy. I had two sessions every day of occupational therapy, physical therapy, and speech therapy. I was discharged about one week later and set up for out-patient therapy sessions and numerous doctor appointments. I enjoyed the sessions and could see improvement daily. I was able to walk with a cane and get around much better. I started to drive again which was tricky at first. My driving scared the life out of my wife—a great carepartner, by the way. She said after a while, "I'll give you one year to recover." I don't know what she meant by that, but whenever she gave me a list of things to do I said to her, "I suffered a stroke, you know."

**"I have come to the realization that a stroke is not just a personal event, but greatly affects the entire family."**

My two sons were also very supportive. One of my sons was able to move home for two months, and that was a great help to both my wife and me. I have come to the realization that a stroke is not just a personal event, but greatly affects the entire family and I realize I could not have gotten through it without my family and friends.

My goal after the stroke was to return to work. However, after six months of therapy I decided to retire early. I had improved greatly but realized my energy level and some problem-solving abilities were still lacking.

Since my stroke and retirement, I have gotten involved with Tai Chi exercise classes once a week and the StrokeWise education program. The Tai Chi has helped a lot with my balance and has taught me some relaxation techniques. I never forgot how good I felt having a peer visitor talk to me in the hospital, so I decided I would like to return the favor. I went to training sessions, and I now volunteer one day a week to visit stroke survivors. I've met a lot of amazing people that have truly been an inspiration. I hope I give back as much as I receive.

❧ ❧

### Learn relaxation techniques.

It's easy to get frustrated when you're learning how to live with your new brain. Relaxation techniques such as Tai Chi, yoga, massage, meditation, and deep breathing exercises can help put your body and mind at ease. Even a quiet moment savoring a delicious cup of coffee or tea can rejuvenate your spirit.

## Tai Chi

Tai Chi is an ancient Chinese form of moving meditation. The series of movements are designed to promote health and well-being. Since the movements are done on both sides of the body, physical and occupational therapists strongly recommend Tai Chi for stroke survivors because it helps with balance, relaxation, and muscle control. The form of Tai Chi most suited to stroke survivors is Tai Chi Chih. This gentle exercise can be done sitting down or standing up, and is easily modified. The group environment provides camaraderie that can be an invaluable help to recovery.

> "Work can take all the energy you have and leave none for anything else."
>
> STROKE THRIVER'S GROUP MEMBER

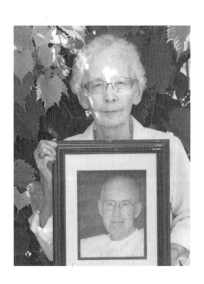

# Keep Coming Back

*by* Donna

Roy never gave up. He kept coming back to therapy, because he recognized that recovery is a lifelong process. Roy had a massive stroke in 1992, which paralyzed his right side, affected much of his speech, and significantly compromised his reading ability. Roy was a MENSA member (an individual with an IQ in the top two percent of the population), and his goal in therapy was to read again and understand the complex content of what he read. In rigorous therapy he rediscovered his ability to read. He tackled up to seven complex magazines a month, including *The Progressive, The Atlantic, Time, The Nation,* and many others. He also read one to three books per week. Reading was Roy's "mental floss" and opened the door to adventure, new knowledge, and improved verbal expression.

Donna, his wife, was his advocate, carepartner, and best friend. She spent time daily exercising his arm and leg and doing everything possible to keep Roy's spirits up. Initially, when Roy couldn't say her name and called their dog, Reggie, a "woof-woof," Donna challenged him to reach his full potential. She credits Roy's persistence to the neurologist who took so much interest in him and kept ordering more therapy during his 13-year recovery process. "Have a strong physician advocate," Donna advises, "one who is there for you throughout the journey."

She also recognizes the impact Roy's therapists had on his progress. "The will for a patient to persevere also depends on the interest, encouragement, insight, and caring of sincerely dedicated professional therapists. Without such compassionate individuals, a patient cannot begin to approach his maximum capability."

Caregiving, especially over so many years, takes its toll. Donna remembers well how Roy's passing "left a big hole in my heart." Many of her own personal health issues needed to be addressed as she processed Roy's passing and attended to her own physical and emotional needs.

What kept this dynamic team afloat was Roy's sense of humor and their ability to openly communicate with each other. "He always maintained a cheerful spirit and a twinkle in his eye. That memory remains bright," Donna says.

※ ※

**Persistence pays off.**
Rehabilitation therapy makes a significant difference in the ongoing recovery process. Roy kept returning to therapy, expecting the highest standards of himself. He was able to regain his ability to read. Research indicates that the brain can form new pathways and enhance skills, regardless of when the stroke occurred.

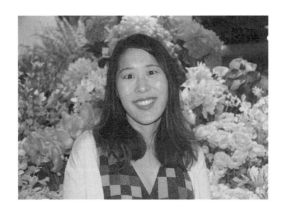

# An Open Window

*by* Anna

They say that when God closes a door, he always opens a window. This is my favorite saying, and I am now able to appreciate what it really means.

My name is Anna. I am 30 years old, and I have a story to tell. I was adopted from Korea when I was four months old. I was brought into a home with wonderful parents and an older sister. I enjoyed my childhood and looked forward to what my future would hold. I graduated from St. Thomas with a Bachelor's Degree in Social Work. I entered the work force with hopes and dreams. At 25, I was hired as a Child Services Social Worker specializing with Native American children and families. I had been doing this for about two years when I became somewhat restless. I was satisfied and challenged, but I felt I needed to find my niche. I had always been interested in health care, so one day I enrolled in prerequisite courses for nursing. I loved it and was doing very well. I applied to the nursing program and was number five on the waiting list. I was nearly done with Anatomy I, with one more month to go, when my life changed dramatically.

On April 15, 2004, at 27 years of age, I had an ischemic stroke. I didn't understand what had happened to me. All I knew was that I was alive, but something was very wrong. I remember crying a lot, especially when I saw my family and friends. I realized I couldn't talk and had difficulty moving my right arm and hand. I spent the next three weeks in the hospital going to speech therapy and occupational therapy.

In speech therapy I had to re-learn my ABCs, simple vocabulary, and how to identify everyday objects. In my mind I recognized what the images were, but I wasn't able to verbalize them. It was so frustrating. It felt like there was a wall in my brain that I couldn't jump over. Right after the stroke, I could say "Mom," "Dad," and "Why," but I couldn't say my boyfriend's name, "Joe." I had to describe him as the big, bald guy. I had to find other words to say what it was I wanted. I had a lot of trouble with polysyllabic words, but luckily my speech therapist introduced a new method that broke down the word. For example, the word "executive" breaks down to "eggs-ec-u-tive." This really worked for me. I still get stuck every now and then with multi-syllable words. It is amazing how many words do not sound like how they are written. I understand how people from other countries have trouble with the English language. Looking back, the tasks I hated most were reading passages aloud and incorporating words into short stories. I now see how it gives my brain a good aerobic exercise.

I had to re-learn how to tie my shoes, cut paper with scissors (they were heavy, sharp, and scary due to my loss of control), write, and figure out first-grade math problems. I worked with large pegs and copied easy designs for coordination. I was shown how to butter bread, put keys in locks, and other cognitive tasks. I often didn't have control of my hand and arm and would knock things over. If I was holding a cup of coffee, I wouldn't even know that the cup was sideways. I called it the "mystery hand." I think I had to find the humor in an otherwise sad condition.

I remember being angry and sad at times. I don't think I realized that my life was going to be so changed. I got frustrated easily and would get mad and cry about things that I used to do so easily. Everything seemed to take me so long, like putting on my seatbelt, unlocking a door, getting dressed, putting make-up on, and spreading butter on toast, all of which looked awkward. There were so many mispronounced words. After a while I was able to laugh about how I said the words. For example, I was at a pond, and I got excited and said, "Look at the dickies" (ducks), "Can I have a Milly?" (a Miller Lite), and my favorite: "I live on Old Shakopoo" (Shakopee). Even now, three years later, I still fumble on words especially when I am tired, stressed, or nervous. Laughter was key for me, and still is.

Right after the stroke, people would say that I would soon be back to doing what I was doing before the stroke. I think I also believed that I would wake up and life would be how it used to be. People would say they couldn't even tell that I had a stroke. I tried to explain to them that conversationally I speak well, minus a few mispronounced words, but my brain inside is affected. I now realize I won't be the same as I used to be, and that is okay.

During the struggles I was going through in my life, I felt blessed and grateful to have had such a strong support system around me. I realized that I wouldn't be where I am today if my parents, sister, friends, co-workers, doctors, and therapists had not been there for me. I believe God sent me all these wonderful people to give me the strength to go on.

I am driving my car again, even though I was told I would never be able to drive. I play cribbage, work jigsaw puzzles and crosswords, and I finally understand Sudoko, which two years ago was foreign to me. I read many books and now write in a journal, which I didn't think I'd be able to do again. I am able to enjoy fishing again, even reel a fish in, and put a minnow on the hook with my affected arm and hand.

Writing this has given me a chance to reexamine my life. I've realized that I still have some sorrow in my heart about losses, changes, and the future. I have decided to seek counseling to work with the emotional part of how my life has changed. Although my prior dreams have deviated, I am hopeful for what will come. "When God closes a door, he opens a window." I am able to see that my window is clearly open. I will end with a quote from Jeremiah 29:11: "For I know the plans I have for you, says the Lord. They are plans for good . . . to give you hope and a future."

> **"Writing this has given me a chance to reexamine my life. I've realized that I still have some sorrow in my heart about the losses, changes, and the future. Although my prior dreams have deviated, I am hopeful for what will come."**

Here is an update from Anna:

My dreams for a new future are coming true. Now, several years after my stroke, the road has taken a new direction now. I started a new job in the social work area. I am still working part-time, but I am hopeful I can get the okay eventually to go back full time. Best of all, I am engaged to be married.

❧ ❧

### Grieve your losses and move forward.

Allowing yourself to journey through the phases of grief is an integral part of processing the losses you experience following brain injury. The challenges you face might include loss of employment, increased financial concerns, changes in body image, issues in your relationships, and loss of friends. Losing the ability to drive can impact your job, social life, and independence.

Well-meaning family and friends sometimes don't understand that you need to grieve even the little things. People tend to minimize daily challenges to try to help you feel better. But it's important that you grieve each thing that you miss, no matter how small. Remember, it can be challenging to work through the fear, anger, denied despair, and guilt without seeing a skilled counselor. As Anna discovered, she needed to seek help so she could address the emotional issues surrounding her stroke. After the counseling, Anna could accept her new brain and move on with her life.

❧ "I have found that counseling can help anxiety, depression, and dissatisfaction with life, even years after the stroke."

STROKE THRIVER'S GROUP MEMBER

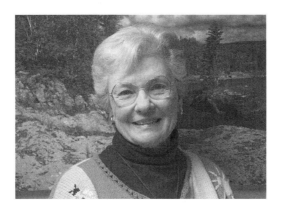

# Ten Guidelines for Writing Your Life Story

*by* Pat

Pat is the author of several books, including *The Book of Positive Quotations for Our Golden Years,* and is on her own courageous communication journey. Pat has primary progressive aphasia, which has affected her ability to speak. Her aphasia was not caused by a stroke.

1. FOCUS
This guidebook already assumes that you are writing this for yourself, first and foremost. Before you begin, or in the early stages of writing, name others you are writing for, such as your children, their children, nephews and nieces, etc. Keep them in mind as you write each story.

2. BE NATURAL
Be yourself. Write like you speak. Tell a story with a beginning,

middle, and end. Let it reflect your personality, and don't worry about a style of writing. Your own voice will emerge as you write.

## 3. BE TRUTHFUL

Whatever you choose to write, let it be the truth. Avoid writing about the way you wish things had been. Write about what actually happened—from your point of view (and be prepared for other points of view from siblings).

## 4. BALANCE

Life is not all bad or all good, so strive to write your life showing views of all the parts of you. You don't want it to become a sterile account of events.

## 5. CONNECT

As you begin to write, many other memories will unfold. Jot them down somewhere to pursue later. As you record these ideas, lists, questions, and the stories themselves, include all the connections you can. Connect past with past, past with present, and past with future. These connections will lead you to a new dimension and appreciation of your own life and heritage. It will connect you to your best self. It will give future generations something to think about.

## 6. FEELINGS

Virginia Wolfe said that too many memoirs record what happened but leave out feelings. It can make the difference in whether your story is boring or interesting. Avoid clichés but use humor to reveal that your life wasn't all serious.

## 7. SENSES

Write about things you can see, hear, feel, smell, taste. Very often your feelings will be connected to one or more of your senses. If you want your readers to really feel what you felt and see what you saw, be sure to describe the scene in which each story takes place.

## 8. TITLE

Begin with a rough draft. Don't expect miracles. Complete your rough draft, then leave it for a day or two. The title is there in your writing. Revise with the title in mind. Limit each story to one page. This is a handy discipline to help you stay focused and cut out useless or flowery words.

## 9. INSPIRATION

Don't wait for inspiration. Write, then inspiration will come. Writing generates writing.

## 10. FREE WRITING

Prime your own pump with 5 to 10 minutes of free writing before each session of writing. Today I feel . . . I remember . . . I wish . . . I was thinking of . . . I was surprised . . .

Pat shares her own poetry in a series of haikus. Haiku is a form of Japanese poetry consisting of five syllables in the first line, seven syllables in the second line, and five syllables in the third line.

## HAIKU

Nuthatch spreads his wings
And fluffs his feathers around
He was showing off.

Nuthatch, Chickadee
Waiting in line for breakfast—
What are they thinking?

November is gray
Like my mind is going to
Mysterious gray.

Snowing at the end
Of December – what lovely
Sight – glory to God

Easter is a time
Of hope, solid stream of God's
Presence in our hearts

**Write your own story.**
You don't have to be a writer to write your own story. The key to unlocking mental blocks begins with jotting a word or idea down on paper and letting the creativity flow. Use Pat's guidelines, and you'll be surprised at what you can do. Or try writing a haiku.

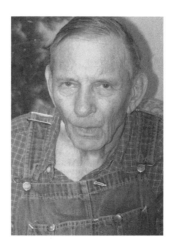

# A Part of Growing Up

*by* Carroll

Carroll had his stroke in August, 2007. When he began therapy, he was not able to write more than two or three short, incomplete sentences. When asked to write about a slice of his life for a speech-therapy assignment, Carroll shared this touching story.

I was born in Cass County, in the state of Minnesota, on January 20, 1928. I lived on a small farm about a mile west of what used to be a small village called Ellis.

The village of Ellis had a general store and a post office, two churches, and a country school. There were other buildings, too, but now all those buildings are gone except the country school.

The day I was born it was too bad weather for the doctor to get there, but my great aunt was a midwife, a Danish woman, and she came, and I was born at my home.

We moved to a place a mile south of there and lived there until 1934. The mailman came by our place, only we didn't call it "the mail man," we called it "the stage." A dozen years before that, they brought the mail with horses and a stagecoach. All the roads weren't in yet, so they followed the trails that had been made before. The round trip was 40 miles and must have taken a long day with a team of faster horses.

Mother came down with tuberculosis, and she went to the sanitarium. She was there about six months. Her mother—and her mother's brothers and sisters—pretty much died from tuberculosis. I remember going to see her once, but I couldn't go near. I remember she was standing at the window of the Sanitarium looking out at us, and we looked at her across the field as she stood by a window. Before she came home, or we came home, my father fumigated the house. My mother was sickly for years after that, but we boys were healthy. Mom recovered, and we appreciated that she lived to be 86.

The first time a doctor saw me was when I took a physical for the army when I was 18 years old.

In 1933 I started country school, which was one-and-a-quarter miles away. My brother and I walked to school. All went well for a few weeks, and then my brother got sick in school and cried all the way home. They found out he had scarlet fever, so that was the end of going to school for a while. They came and put a quarantine on our house. We couldn't leave. All three of us boys had scarlet fever, and when we got over it we moved to the place that we have now. Our house was a granary. We had to make it a home we could live in. We had to build the buildings we would need before winter for the shelter of the animals and poultry. Dad had to get the feed up for the winter. We children were young, but there was always something for us to do, like get wood up, work in the fields, and herd cattle.

In August another brother came, and that made four of us. In the summer, our grandmother (my father's mother) was killed in an automobile accident, so there was a grave to dig. Many tears were shed. I will always remember her love for her flower garden and how we would run on the paths.

**"Frustration decreases in direct proportion to positive action."**

They did all the farm work with horses, and things were a lot different then than they are now. When we went to school it was a two-mile walk each way, but that was good for us. If we wanted to get home faster, we would run instead of walk. We did the work from lamp or lantern light.

We learned how to work in the house, cook, milk cows by hand, etc. Through all of life we were close, because we stood our ground and loved.

Carroll also offers his advice for stroke recovery:

- Read, read, read.

- Talk, talk, talk.

- Write, write, write. ("If I needed a word I thought I should write—when I'm holding the pen—I think about words, and if I can't spell them, I look them up in the dictionary. Suddenly I can spell it next time because I've looked it up.")

- Look up. Reach up. Lift up. Cheer up. Never give up.

- You never get bored when you use your imagination.

- Frustration decreases in direct proportion to positive action.

- Life is a big school, and you never graduate. You have to have heartaches, so that you can get away from yourself and look at people differently. You can learn from others.

- Names of people from the past come back because you use your mind. You must put your mind to work. Use your mind or lose it.

- When you get with other people, you get your mind off of yourself. (Carroll plays guitar every Saturday at the Senior Center. "I sit and talk to people.")

❧ ❧

**Read, talk, write.**
Practice communicating by making it enjoyable. Read stories that you find interesting. Talk to your friends, neighbors, and family about what's happening in their lives. Write about things that inspire you. Carroll wrote about his childhood, and in the process called up beautiful memories of that time.

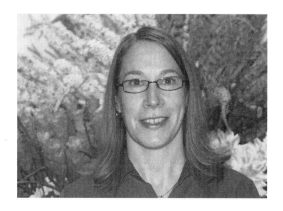

# My Life After a Stroke

*by* Jill

Jill had a stroke when she was 38 years old, resulting in both aphasia and apraxia. Her speech was initially full of sound substitutions and mispronounced words, especially as the length of the message increased. Jill started her recovery by relearning to write her own name and simple words. Later, she was asked to turn in a story as an assignment in speech therapy, and she persevered for a month to write it by hand.

It's challenging to talk and write and read. Numbers are difficult. You take all these things for granted before you have a stroke. When I had the stroke, I couldn't talk or move my right side. It was frustrating. Now it is seven months later, and I'm learning to talk, walk, write, and read. Numbers aren't as difficult as before. One strategy for numbers is counting on my fingers, so I know the number. I discovered that if I see the number by counting on my fingers, then my brain has a connection with the number. For me, if I see the number, then it makes sense. I've discovered that I am a visual person.

Writing was confusing, because I didn't know how to order the words in the sentence. Now I write every day, and sentences are easier. It takes time, but it's worth it.

Before I had the stroke, I was an administrative assistant. I supported three vice presidents, three assistant vice presidents, and three associates. It was a hard and sometimes very stressful job. Now I'm working toward a new career by volunteering and working with a vocational counselor.

I think my stroke was a blessing in disguise. I'm forced to think about life, and maybe there is something new to do. I cry sometimes, and I feel sorry for myself. One minute your brain is doing fine, and the next minute your brain is not the same. That is a harsh reality to accept. I'm learning that you must have a positive outlook in life.

> "I think my stroke was a blessing in disguise. I'm forced to think about life, and maybe there is something new to do."

This handwritten sample illustrates the major progress that Jill has made in her writing ability. Practice makes progress.

It is two years since my stroke and I'm still improving everyday. Im 100% better physically. I garden, walk, ride my bike, take the stairs at home and when I volunteer. This summer I even climbed Bear Butte in Sturgis, SD. In eleven months of volunteering I have increased my stamina from 4 to 16 hours per week. I still have some trouble with communication, numbers, and letters. I think I will always have trouble with this. If I keep interacting with people, work on writing and reading, I will continue to improve.

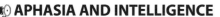

**APHASIA AND INTELLIGENCE**

People who have aphasia can get very frustrated when trying to communicate. They can't form the words they want to say or understand all of what's being said to them. They want to say something and know what it is, but it just won't come out the right way. A common misconception of speech challenges after a stroke is that intelligence is decreased. But aphasia does not affect intelligence. You are still as smart as you were before the stroke, but you may have a hard time getting words out.

**Make communication easier.**

Tips for family and friends of people who have aphasia:

- Stand where you can be seen.

- If there's more than one person in the room, speak one at a time.

- Avoid background noise, such as TV or radio.

- Use a normal tone of voice.

- Use short, simple sentences and pause between thoughts.

- Ask yes-or-no questions.

- Wait 10 to 20 seconds for the answer to a question, and don't interrupt the process.

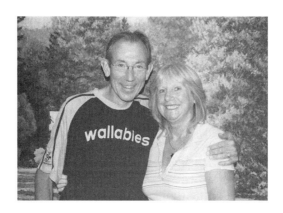

## A Reason for Hope

*by* Dee, as communicated through her husband, Steve

On December 9, 2006, I had a ruptured aneurysm, resulting in a cerebral hemorrhage. This was followed by three brain surgeries, a heart attack, and a severe stroke on the left side of my brain. Based on brain CTs and MRIs, doctors predicted that I would not be able to talk or move my right arm or leg, due to the stroke.

I immediately showed I could move my right side, the day after the stroke. I squeezed my husband's hand, and, when my sons arrived at the hospital, I gave them a big hug with both arms.

When I was discharged from the hospital, I could not talk, write, or type. My ability to speak is slowly progressing. I have been in out-patient speech and occupational therapy for six weeks and am making steady progress. I can read well and understand what others say when they talk to me. I can answer yes-or-no questions and can usually get my point across even when I can't say a specific word.

I learned a few weeks ago that when I couldn't say a word, I could write down a word or two to get the point across. For example, if I'm asking my husband about a certain person, I just write their name on a piece of paper. This has worked so well that I have paper and pencils with me all the time—at meals, in the car with my husband, or when going out with my girlfriends.

My husband has also created lists to help me make choices. For example, if I want to go out to a restaurant, he shows me a list with my 20 favorite places, and I just point to the one I want. This also helps to facilitate communication. When you think about it, the words you speak are only a small part of what you communicate. Your body language, gestures, writing, voice tone and inflection—all help you communicate.

With continued therapy, I am confident of being able to talk normally. And I am motivated to show the doctors that I can do what they thought would be impossible. With faith and the right attitude, anything is possible.

**"I am motivated to show the doctors that I can do what they thought would be impossible. With faith and the right attitude, anything is possible."**

Dee's husband Steve and her sons Tyler and Shane recalled what it was like to watch Dee undergo three brain surgeries and experience a heart attack and stroke.

Dee was in the hospital for eight weeks, 18 days in intensive care. Interestingly, she doesn't remember any of it (which probably is good). But we remember those days in detail, especially when the medical staff told us Dee might not make it. So when Dee finally came home, she knew she had to heal, but she didn't understand how sick she was. When we told her how much she had improved, she really didn't see it. She just knew she couldn't get her words out and that frustrated her.

We all can see the gradual progress Dee is making in speaking words and sentences. Two weeks ago, Dee learned to say, "How are you?" She was so excited that she said it to everyone she met in the next week. In fact, she still says it over and over.

Last night, Dee and I had the evening alone. We left our Sunday church service at 6:00 p.m., and Dee told me she wanted to go out for a special dinner. With her paper and pen, she wrote a couple words that I was able to decipher—Campiello—a favorite restaurant we had not eaten at since Dee's accident. We had a two-hour, romantic dinner with constant conversation. And, while Dee cannot pronounce all of her words yet, I did not feel at any disadvantage when talking. On the contrary, perhaps the conversation was even deeper than before because we each concentrate more. We had fun and a fabulous dinner.

**Use a variety of strategies to communicate.**
Spoken words are only a part of communication. In addition to the 25 to 30 phrases Dee can say, she uses gestures, facial expressions, and written words to communicate with her family and friends. Dee and her husband have come up with creative communication tools, including the list of their favorite restaurants. To challenge herself, Dee regularly attends an aphasia conversation group and has telephone conversations with her family in Australia.

> "Nothing a healthcare professional can say is as healing as the words of someone in the same boat."
>
> STROKE THRIVER'S GROUP LEADER

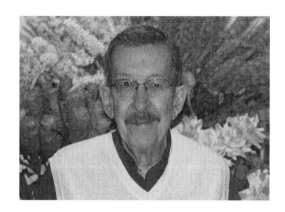

# Ivan and His Dog
*by* Ivan

My name is Ivan.

Years ago, when we (that's myself, my wife, and our first four children) lived in our first house, I would stay up late and watch TV. My wife Darlene and the kids would all go up to bed.

One night a movie starring Boris Karloff came on—I think it had to do with Frankenstein's monster or a werewolf or Dracula.

I was watching with our dog, Yanoush, at my feet.

Boris Karloff's mother was played by Maria Ouspenskaya. When his mother left the room, she said to her son (Boris K.) "Yanoush, you should go to bed." He replied, "I will," and said to his dog (a great Dane), "Come along, Ivan."

Needless to say, I laughed out loud. Ivan and his dog, Yanoush, watching Yanoush and his dog, Ivan.

Ivan contracted mononucleosis encephalitis in 1980. In 1991, he had a heart attack. Six years later he suffered a ruptured aortal aneurysm. After that he experienced a small stroke and another heart attack. "I'm not sure, but everyone else says I am a miracle person. I suppose it's because I've been at death's door so many times. I myself think it's because the Lord is giving me more chances to shape up," Ivan says.

**Laugh for your health.**

Laughter is an integral part of the therapy process. It results in healthy heart-to-heart connections and acts as "mental floss" to the mind. Ivan's story about his dog showed that he still looks for humor in his daily life. Even though he's been through horrendous experiences, he still is able to find humor in them. How can you bring more laughter into your life?

**"Hearty laughter is a good way to jog internally without having to go outdoors."**

NORMAN COUSINS

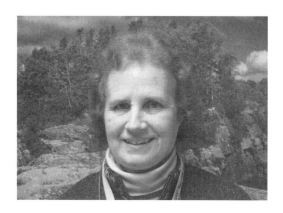

# Doing Things Differently

*by* Beth

Charles Swindoll said that life is 10 percent what happens to you and 90 percent what you do with what happens to you. I think this maxim especially applies to life after stroke. Having a stroke is devastating. In my case, the stroke disrupted my career as a law librarian and my avocation as a musician. It left me paralyzed on the right side of my body and it affected my memory, my voice, and my fortitude. However, I eventually realized that I couldn't just sit around and feel sorry for myself. It wasn't impossible to do things anymore; I just needed to do things differently.

For instance, I can't walk like I used to walk. I go very slowly. Sometimes I joke that if I went any slower I'd go backwards. On the other hand, because I move so slowly I pay more attention to who and what is around me. I also can't carry a laundry basket and run quickly down to the washing machine, like I used to. I now push a cart with the laundry basket on top of it. But, once a week, I get the clothes clean.

I can't sing like I used to sing. I used to direct or sing alto in church and community choirs. Sometimes I sang solos. Now I have a hard time singing the tenor part. My voice is not very strong. However, singing with the church choir is still rewarding. I've met new people. I have a different director's perception of how a piece should be interpreted. And the creative side of me is still stimulated to relay a message to others in song.

To my great regret, I can't work as a law librarian anymore. Although I finally can once again understand what needs to be done to run a library, I don't have the strength to work regularly or even to drive across town to work each day. On the other hand, I've found a new outlet for my ideas—writing. I am challenged to put my thoughts down on paper, and to accurately express my feelings.

Mind you, I haven't accepted all these changes in my life without a struggle. Just as I had to break my arm three times as a child before I learned my first lesson in patience, I tried to live life as I used to live it—before I finally realized that I've been given a second chance to improve upon my life. A stroke causes a lot of changes. What's important is how I deal with those changes.

"I haven't accepted all these changes in my life without a struggle. Just as I had to break my arm three times as a child before I learned my first lesson in patience, I tried to live life as I used to live it—before I finally realized that I've been given a second chance to improve upon my life."

**Find a new way to do what you love.**

At first, many brain injury survivors feel they are on a detour and will soon return to the same life they were living before. At some point, most realize they are actually on a new road. But as Beth discovered with her singing, this new road has its own rewards. She returned to activities she used to do and still found pleasure in them, even though she couldn't participate in the same way as before. Take a look at what you did before your life changed, and see how you can still do what you love in a different way. What new things can you try?

**Sing to bring harmony to the heart and strength to the body.**

Singing is a great communication and respiratory-strengthening strategy. Even though your voice may change following a stroke, singing is encouraged because of the wide range of therapeutic benefits, including increased rhythm and flow of speech, improved articulation and voicing, and stronger respiration and vocal folds. Singing is a right-hemisphere activity, but it seems to unlock words from the left hemisphere. Singing the words to your favorite songs can help inspire more confidence in your speech.

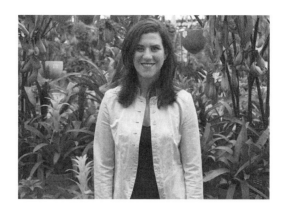

## Looking to the Horizon

*by* Tiffany

Have you ever stopped to think how a life-threatening experience could make a lasting impression on the remainder of your life?

If someone would have asked me that question a year ago, I would have undoubtedly given them a vague response, with little to no emotion involved. However, now I will never be able to answer that question in the same way, as I am a stroke survivor. I had a left-temporal hemorrhagic stroke on October 4, 2006.

Up until that date, I had everything I ever dreamed of, including success with my professional career, great relationships with family and friends, and the aspirations to attend law school in fall, 2007, to become an attorney. What more could a healthy 26-year-old ask for? I was truly blessed and knew that bigger and better things were on the horizon.

My 26th birthday was an enjoyable day; however, it was evident to everyone that I was not feeling or acting like myself. I woke up on October 4, at 3:00 a.m., not able to read, write, speak, or, most importantly, dial my cell phone to contact the emergency room. Thankfully, my boyfriend at the time had spent the night and discovered me sitting in my living room with a confused look on my face. He immediately knew something was terribly wrong and contacted the hospital.

**"One of the greatest outcomes of this experience is that I have become a spokesman for stroke. I enjoy educating and teaching the community on the subject of stroke. I would not trade my new life for the world. "**

After the stroke my dreams were crushed, because my diagnosis and prognosis were both grim. I did not think, based on everything I had heard about my medical status, that I would ever be able to meet my goals and turn my dreams into reality. I had extreme deficits in all areas and was barely able to say hello or do simple math, such as 2 + 2.

However, a miracle has occurred with the hope and inspiration of my physicians, therapists, family, and friends. Today I am well on my way to full recovery from my stroke. I am at approximately 95 percent recovery; however, I still experience some aphasia when speaking verbally or communicating in writing.

One of the greatest outcomes of this experience is that I have become a spokesman for stroke. I enjoy educating and teaching the community on the subject of stroke. I would not trade my new life for the world, and I want to say thanks for giving me a new and fresh perspective on life.

I went back to work and succeeded in the role I had before my stroke. Nearly two years after my stroke, I was promoted to an even more challenging position in my company. It's a position that takes more organization, thinking, traveling, and working outside of my comfort zone. It makes me feel great. I was due for a challenge.

My stroke brought everything to a screeching halt. When I was able to recover and go back to work, it was my motivation to progress faster than ever before. I've never been happier, because before my stroke I took my speaking and writing for granted. Now, I appreciate the value of being independent and growing personally and professionally on a daily basis.

❧ ☙

**Use your experience to help others.**
Speaking about your experience with stroke can offer crucial inspiration, support, and education while giving you an opportunity to enrich your own life. Taking action rids survivors of the sense of helplessness so common after a traumatic event and provides a sense of accomplishment that builds self-esteem and confidence.

> ❧ "Exercise ideas: Tai Chi, walk daily, silver sneakers
> at a health club, recumbent elliptical machine,
> walk up and down stairs every day."
>
> STROKE THRIVER'S GROUP MEMBER

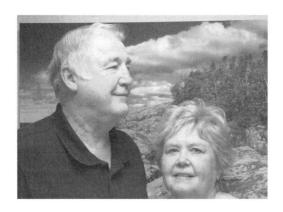

# Roads and Signs

*by* Marvin and Madalyn (the "M&Ms")

Life is a well-traveled road. The longer you live, the more you realize it is not always smooth. It has hills to climb, unexpected curves to maneuver, bumps that slow you down, and ruts that can throw you off track. There are also signs to guide you that sometimes we ignore, later causing us to suffer the consequences. And so it was with us.

At age 22 we had college degrees and a marriage license in hand, all in one exciting week. We were ready to travel down this planned, "smooth" road together. We had jobs, moved several times due to three years in the military, purchased a lovely home, and settled down to raise our three sons. We started a business together, then purchased another; Marv designed, developed, and patented a lift for people with disabilities that was installed on vans. Life was challenging and busy, but life was good.

After our children were educated, married, and left home, we remained in our original home, certain to retire there and take it easy. But in the dead of winter, while we were away from home, our house started on fire—and before anyone noticed it, the windows blew out, and flames were shooting high in the sky. We were notified by our dear neighbors. In disbelief, we rushed home to find fire trucks lining the lane and a crowd of neighbors and friends all trying to help. We watched as 45 years of memories seemed to fade into the distance. How could this happen? We mourned the loss of our dear April, a golden retriever and her best friend, Molly Dolly, the cat. At the time, all our sons were out of town on business, but they scurried home, one even from Japan, while their families surrounded us and took us in. For us, this was not a curve in the road—it seemed like a dead end. Why hadn't we seen the sign? Was there even a sign? And why us?

As the days passed, we came to realize that we still had each other, our family, and our friends. They all had been so generous to us. True thanksgiving to God for what we had left took away our sadness, and we began to rebuild our lives again. Eventually, the remains of our home were hauled away, and we purchased a town home in a neighboring suburb. Selecting new furniture and, in essence, re-establishing our home in newlywed fashion was both an overwhelming and satisfying experience. Life was back on track again, and it was good.

Some challenges remained. Insurance payments were slow, paperwork was taking more time than usual, and several trees needed to be felled and removed at our original home site. It was on a warm July day that Marv decided to trim a tree instead of waiting for help to arrive. He climbed up on a storage shed and, while cutting a limb, he lost his balance and fell approximately 10 feet onto the concrete below, with chainsaw in hand. Lying unconscious for nearly an hour before being found by a friend, he was rushed in an ambulance to the trauma center. We found Marv in intensive care and unresponsive, with a broken back, shoulder, and ribs and a severe brain injury. As we stood by his bed, we couldn't help but wonder: Was this the end of the road? Pastor Dan came, and we prayed fervently that somehow the road would continue for Marv. Our hours turned into days, but we remained hopeful that this, too, would pass.

**"Being extremely independent all his life, Marv found depending on Madalyn for help difficult. "**

Then, early in the morning of the fourth day, Madalyn leaned down and whispered "I love you" in Marv's ear, and his eyes opened. It was only for a few seconds, but it gave us renewed hope and much joy. Yes! Just maybe this road will continue. Yes! Even bumpy was okay with us now.

Eventually Marv was moved out of intensive care into another well-guarded area. Pain was a constant reminder of his injuries, although the mind has a wonderful way of erasing these discomforts. He seemed content to sleep his life away, even when his sleep was interrupted with endless x-rays and evaluations. The normal routine of life had to be relearned, so Marv moved into the rehab center. Standing, walking, balancing, and eating were all challenges. Things that he used to do unconsciously now took all the concentration he could muster to accomplish. He was mildly frustrated at not being "normal," but managed to maintain a healthy attitude to those who were servicing his needs.

Then came the big day to go home. Watching the daily routine of others was a bit overwhelming for Marv. His life had become slow, and he just wanted to sleep. Granted, he needed rest, but sleep also helped him to deal with his situation—or perhaps *not* deal with it. Being extremely independent all his life, Marv found depending on Madalyn for help difficult. When she was at her part-time job, he felt alone, and he toyed with the idea that he could end this dependence with just one gunshot. At least then he would no longer be a burden on his family. But the constant love and concern of Madalyn and his family was a road sign that he recognized this time. It provided encouragement, guidance, and direction for him. Turn right Marv, turn right. This is not the end of the road. He couldn't forget it. He began to see that taking his own life was not his decision to make.

Marv continued to do his best, and after several months at home he entered rehab again. He found the therapists to be kind, encouraging, helpful, and experienced. His broken shoulder now works well again, and his thinking patterns have improved. The therapists taught him to keep track of his progress on paper, so he can look back and see that he has come a long way. He has learned that being organized is imperative to his recovery. He is still working on this.

So life does go on. It is ours to enjoy. The road is not entirely smooth, and it is different than it was, but it has its pleasant moments. Each day is a gift from God, and again life is good.

❧ ❧

### Know the signs of depression.
Approximately one out of two stroke survivors experience depression, and many express suicidal thoughts. In fact, stroke survivors have a higher rate of depression than individuals with several physical injuries and disability from other causes. Marv's desire to sleep away the days was a symptom of his wish to avoid facing his feelings. It can be difficult to distinguish the fatigue common after a brain injury from depression that

needs to be treated. Depression can be related to grief over the many losses associated with brain injury, including loss of independence, changes in body image and relationships, difficulties with communication, and dealing with physical disabilities. It is also thought to sometimes be tied to the chemical changes in the brain caused by the injury. If you experience any symptoms of depression, get help from your doctor or a mental-health professional.

**SYMPTOMS OF DEPRESSION**
- Persistent sad or anxious mood

- Feelings of hopelessness, pessimism, guilt, worthlessness, or helplessness

- Loss of interest or pleasure in hobbies and activities that were once enjoyed

- Fatigue, decreased energy, or a sense of being slowed down

- Difficulty concentrating, remembering, or making decisions

- Insomnia, early-morning awakening, or oversleeping

- Appetite and / or weight changes

- Restlessness or irritability

- Thoughts of death or suicide, or suicide attempts

“Medication for depression is helpful. That was a surprise.”

STROKE THRIVER'S GROUP MEMBER

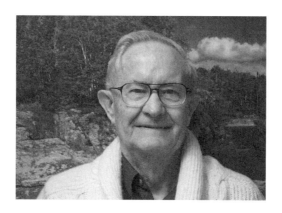

# In a Day's Work

*by* Harry S.

After leaving a daughter's home in Bozeman, Montana, to return home to Bloomington, Minnesota, I was suddenly unable to drive my car. My wife, Sally, took me to the clinic back at Bozeman. The doctor thought I needed a heart specialist, which was not available in Bozeman. What a gorgeous view I had that late afternoon and evening, looking down from a helicopter at 12,000 feet over the mountains as we traveled 200 miles to a hospital in Billings, Montana.

When I awoke from surgery, my nurse offered me water. I could drink and swallow, and she said, "Wonderful! You are lucky because so many cannot swallow after a stroke." So you can see, my stroke wasn't too serious—though I could not name my wife or daughter for two days. During our drive home, I got to know them really well.

Many tests at the hospital near my home showed that I was a good candidate for rehab therapy that would reteach me how to read, write, count money, and write checks.

I retired from volunteering in the hospital print shop and began volunteering instead at Bridging, a charitable-services center in Bloomington, Minnesota. This company provides for families who have a home but nothing in it to make it a real home. We give the families mattresses, kitchen equipment, chairs, lamps, sofas, bedding, glassware, utensils, and dressers—about all they need to make a home a home.

My first work there was to repair anything made of wood that could be usable. Then I was switched to the electric shop. This work allows me to give help to people who need it. Doing this helps me to be active—walking, toting heavy lamps, talking to many different people, and lunching with friends. All this keeps me using my mind and hands and gets me back some of the dexterity I had before the stroke. In spite of the stroke, I'm still able to work, be active, and feel good about myself.

❧ ☙

**Discover ways you can stay active.**
Whether you return to an old job, find a new one, or volunteer, find ways to keep engaged with the world. Like Harry, you'll find that working or volunteering can help you heal physically and emotionally. Adding structure to your day and week can actually help with the fatigue common to survivors. You have a reason to get going and the company of people who can stimulate your thoughts and energy.

❧ **"Challenge yourself to do something different every day."**
STROKE THRIVER'S GROUP MEMBER

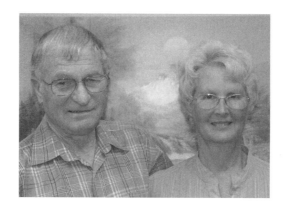

## It Takes Two

*by* Ann

Roger's wife, Ann, remembers the night of her husband's stroke.

Roger turned on the TV to catch the news. I told him I was going to the barn to check the horses. I was gone 20 minutes, and when I came back, Roger was just standing at the sink like he was looking out the window. But he didn't seem to notice I'd come back to the house. I asked if he was okay, and he didn't answer. I thought he didn't hear me. When I walked over and asked again if he was okay, I knew he wasn't. He just looked at me, and I couldn't understand his words at all.

Roger had had heart bypass surgery in 1998, but I knew this wasn't his heart. I wasn't positive, but I guessed he'd had a stroke, and I knew I needed to get him to the hospital. I called the hospital and got a recording, so I got him into the car. He had no trouble walking, but I couldn't understand his speech. For a half a minute before we left for the hospital, his speech was normal, but he didn't know what had happened. Then the garbled words came again. I knew he knew what I was talking about, because he could shake his head yes or no. He had a bad headache on the front left side. We drove to a town 25 miles away. Roger held on to my arm. He was confused by what had happened and was scared.

We spent Sunday night until morning in ICU. It took until noon before Roger could say his name, and by Monday night at 8:00 p.m. he could say Ann correctly. He knew who his kids were and knew their names, but couldn't say them. He was exhausted on Monday; it had been a long night. He was able to do the mobility checks okay. It was the words that would not come.

Tuesday we moved to the stroke floor. Roger was able to move around and could go for walks, but his speech was confused. It was hard to explain things to him. When he ate meals, he ate so fast. I had to keep telling him to slow down, so unusual for him. He normally doesn't hurry through a meal. He knew the kids and seemed to recall what was going on, but just couldn't tell us. I thought I would bring some pictures from home and see if he could tell me what they were and what was going on in the pictures. He could. Then I had him show the pictures to Pam, his nurse, and he told her about them. We did occupational therapy and speech therapy. Remembering was a challenge. It still is, but it's getting better. When Roger gets tired, he really has to search for words. When I brought him home, I wondered what I could do to help him the most. I taught him to use the ruler again, and we did some easy projects. It was easier to go back to what was familiar and to start there.

Roger's brother, Allen, came two weeks after Roger had the stroke. Allen was a tremendous help to Roger's therapy. We would all three go to the speech-therapy sessions, and Allen would come home and continue the session with Roger all day long. They would talk about so many things. Allen didn't let Roger cut his sentences short or substitute words. Allen spent a week with us, helping and contributing so much to Roger's recovery. I really believe that at that time Roger's brain changed the most, because he had his own personal coach for speech therapy. He was like a kid in school. He would learn something in therapy and come home and practice for the week. We owe Allen so much and can't thank him enough for his contribution to Roger's miraculous recovery.

It's still hard for Roger to spell words. He looks most of them up, but it's hard because he's not always close on the spelling. To put his thoughts on paper is very hard. It just doesn't flow. It's getting better, but he is exhausted from the task. Still, he doesn't give up. Just recently, he began typing stories and e-mails.

I went to all the therapy sessions to see how I could help, because I knew it would take a lot of repetition to make life smooth again. Roger's physical health is pretty stable now. His blood pressure and cholesterol are where the doctors want them. He is active and can do most of the things he did before. It just takes longer, and he has to think it through longer. Working with his hands seemed to be good therapy. He could make things and fix things again and was doing something he knew how to do. Writing his thoughts on paper and getting it to flow is a struggle, but that, too, will come.

We appreciate all the help in therapy. It's going to take some time and more work, but we'll get there.

**Work together.**

Your spouse or carepartner is an important member of your care team, who can help you reach your recovery goals. Husband and wife roles change following brain injury, so it's important that you talk to each other about your needs. For family members, meeting the challenging needs of the survivor requires creativity, flexibility, and the ability to discover the humor and gifts within the frustrating moments. With Ann's help, Roger has returned to farming, gardening, and home-maintenance projects. Ann and Roger have demonstrated what is achievable when couples work together in the therapy process.

❧ **"Talk with people who care about you."**

STROKE THRIVER'S GROUP MEMBER

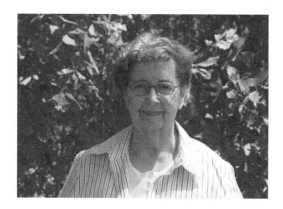

# The Importance of Perseverance

*by* Eleanor

I have enjoyed relatively good health most of my life. My husband and I have spent our winters in Texas for many years. Our lives have been active. But in September, 2006, I found myself on the floor of my bathroom unable to help myself up. My husband had already called 911. The response was immediate.

I remember asking the ambulance driver, "Did I have a TIA?"* His reply was that I had had a major stroke. It was important to arrive at the hospital within a three-hour time period for possible treatment.

It was agreed that I should be moved to a rehab center for therapy. I was determined from the start to work hard—to do my best. I was very motivated. Therapy, therapy, therapy.

---

* TIA stands for "transient ischemic attack"—stroke symptoms that go away on their own, often within minutes or hours. Do not ignore these symptoms. Seek medical care immediately, as a TIA puts you at risk for a major stroke. It is a warning sign.

I was able to drive the car and care for myself. All was going well until, one day, I suddenly had a difficult time communicating with my husband. He immediately called 911, and I was taken to the hospital again.

I felt fine, but the words would not come out of my mouth. I was experiencing another stroke. This time I was suffering from aphasia. Nothing was making sense. I knew what I wanted to say, but it wouldn't come out. Once again, I immediately knew that I needed to concentrate on therapy.

The most important thing for me was that I had to persevere. My hard work is paying off. I am able to do crossword puzzles, and I plan to work constantly to continue to improve.

Here are some of Eleanor's tips for other stroke survivors:

- Talk with friends on the phone, through e-mail, and in social settings. Don't be shy.

- Use the dictionary. Look up words. Read the newspaper. Skim it, read headlines, and pick up ideas and words.

- Crossword puzzles in the paper are excellent therapy. Begin with simple ones and go to more complex ones.

- When you begin reading, start simply with poetry, children's books such as Dr. Seuss, and greeting cards. Reading out loud jump-starts the brain. Do it often, and you will experience improved speech.

- Take advantage of plays, concerts, movies, and other community events. They provide conversational nuggets and are good.

- Play the piano, sing, tap out the beat, and dance, because these activities wake up the body and brain simultaneously.

- Use your experience to reach out, help, and encourage others.

- Don't give up. I've learned now to express my thoughts by being persistent. The more you talk, the better your speech gets. All my friends let me talk, and I feel very comfortable that I can do that. If I can't say a word, they tell me to go ahead and try it. I then get more confidence that I can make sense.

❧ ☙

**You are still the same person.**
One of the most important aspects of stroke recovery is to remember that you are the same person you've always been. You will feel better doing the things you enjoy, even if in slightly altered ways. Music has always been important to Eleanor and has contributed to her recovery. Retreating from your loved ones and isolating yourself from them is not conducive to a healthy and whole life. Your family members and close friends want to continue to be involved in your life and your activities. Get back into the world again.

❧ "Finding a good listener is a treasure."
STROKE THRIVER'S GROUP MEMBER

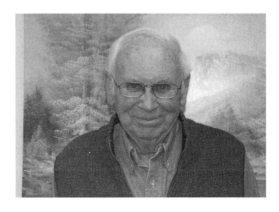

## Harry Truman Used My Pen

*by* Russell

In 1956 I was a passenger on a propeller airplane departing from Minneapolis, bound for Kansas City. A stewardess informed me that I would be having a very special seat partner: President Harry Truman. He came onto the airplane with bodyguards and sat down right next to me. He was just as jolly and pleasant as he could possibly be. We talked. He shared that he was going to Italy to talk to generals who "needed to be talked to."

I was carrying an expensive Parker 51 gold-capped pen in my pocket, and President Truman didn't have a pen. He borrowed mine to give his autograph to everyone who requested it. We landed at many small towns. With each stop, the stewardess would come and say, "President Truman, there are an awful lot of people who want to see you." He would then reach up, get his big hat from the rack above his seat, go to the door, wave his cowboy hat, and laugh. Each time we landed, he would put on his hat, wave to the crowd, and return to his seat, putting his hat into the luggage compartment. He was such a nice person—pleasant and full of smiles.

After a two-hour flight, we prepared for the final landing. I noticed my gold-tipped Parker pen in his pocket. I hesitated to say it but I did, "President Truman, may I have my pen back please?" He laughed, took my pen out of his pocket, and gave it back to me. To this day I still have my pen and President Truman's autograph.

❦ ❦

**To improve fluency, talk about your life experiences.**
Russell, his two daughters, and his speech pathologist collaborated on this story. At treatment onset, he would have groped to speak a story of this complexity. It took him 50 minutes to sequence all the details, and he scored his speech to be a 10 on a scale of one to 10.

Talking about life experiences can improve your speaking skills. Family members are encouraged to talk about past memories and to use familiar objects, such as family photo albums, war medals, sports trophies, county fair ribbons, and other meaningful memorabilia to stimulate conversation.

When information is written down, retention of that information jumps to more than 50 percent. Only a tiny percentage is retained when the message is only heard. Further improvement in memory is marked when the sequence of events is then retold to another. Russell used all of these strategies. He was then able to spontaneously share this story from memory and in perfect sequence at the Life in Bloom aphasia group.

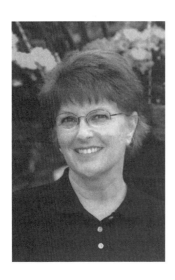

## Signs of New Life

*by* Vicki

This is a story of my experience with **traumatic brain injury** (TBI). It is a story of despair and fear, loneliness and survival, and, finally, hope and peace.

My name is Vicki, and this is what happened to me twenty-seven years ago. I was a passenger in a semi-trailer truck in the early morning of May 1, 1980. My then-husband drove through a red light, causing an accident with another semi-trailer.

Most of my right side was hurt. Worst of all was the severe head wound to my right-front forehead, just above my eye. The details of my injuries were exacerbated by the fact that I was six months pregnant.

I spent approximately three weeks in a coma. I have almost no memory of what happened during that first month, except that I knew my knitting needles were in the truck and wished someone would get them for me. I knew I was pregnant. I also knew that so many people kept asking me questions. I do remember a lot of anger with this "question and answer" game. I really did not feel like telling anyone my name. I was annoyed that so many people were staring at me, when my eyes were usually swollen shut, and I really did not care who "they" were. Finally I told them I recognized Terry, my sister's boyfriend, just to finish the game.

I have often wondered if getting so angry with this challenge, and many more challenges in the next years, is exactly the reason that I survived. I was forced to recognize someone, speak, and respond. The last decades have been full of such attempts at regaining skills and abilities. Some have been successful attempts, and all have been difficult, even frustrating.

Perhaps my first huge successful challenge was the delivery of my son, Andrew, healthy and strong, three months later. The delivery was surgical—and worth every difficult month of recovery.

Surviving until my son was born was a challenge in itself. I suffered from seizures and deep despair. I was isolated in a rural setting, with little help. My husband was not supportive. There were a couple of times when I nearly gave up. I was so weak, so alone, and so helpless. I stayed alive from the sheer will to give my baby a chance at life.

Through this experience, I learned I had to take care of myself first. If I had not kept trying, my son would not have survived. Secretly, my plan had been to deliver my son, close my eyes, and die. One look at that gorgeous kid, with his big dark eyes, and dying was no longer a choice. I fought back against every challenge.

My short-term memory was severely affected. I had to search for words that would not come. I could not always remember with whom I had just spoken. I certainly could not remember anything

I had just read. I began to carry small notebooks with me. I posted notes all over my home and by the telephone, to remind me of times, dates, and people. I felt humiliated and afraid.

My long-term memory was intact. I could still play my first piano recital piece. I could still recite, from memory from third grade, "Paul Revere's Ride" by Henry Wadsworth Longfellow. I could still speak and read much of the German and French languages I had studied. I could still read, although not remember a word I had just read. I read the book *Sacajawea,* by Anna Lee Waldo, three times before I could remember anything about the story. There are 1,342 pages.

My brain could do some things and not others. At the same time, part of my brain knew the other parts were not working correctly. Did I think I was crazy? Yes. Many times.

A year after the accident, I left my marriage. This procedure took longer than I had hoped, and my brain injury was used against me in court. Brain injury brings many hurdles, all of them compounding the initial injury. Life can be cruel. I moved on.

June 17, 1981, is a day that will always be like a happy anniversary for me. It was the day I met with a new neurologist. I had decided to change doctors, get some new information, start over, and begin a happier life.

This doctor was smart, caring, and human. Always, he has treated me with respect. He treated me like I had a brain, even when I was not so sure I had one. He has always been on my side through difficult times. Maybe he knew how long-term this recovery would be.

I have been in lots of hospitals. I have had plastic surgery. I found out that my brain had suffered even more damage. Tests were not done when I was pregnant. After Andrew was born I learned that my brain had actually been thrown around within the skull at the time of the accident. This was not great news, but by this time I had lots of practice facing problems.

Has my life with traumatic brain injury been only problematic? Yes and no. There are days when I could categorize my life as wretched and frightening. There are other days when I realize how lucky I am to have survived and, some might say, thrived.

There have also been huge disappointments. I have not been able to have a wonderful professional career. I have worked many part-time or temporary jobs. I have been forced to take days, months, and even years from my working life just to rest and recuperate.

From each of these hard events I have learned. I learned how to use many different computer programs on these jobs, although I cannot look at the screen when images are moving quickly. Such stimuli can cause a seizure. I had time to volunteer at my son's elementary school. I have learned to read again. I have learned to play new and more difficult piano pieces.

I have even learned to relax during hospitalizations, soaking up the care and concern from wonderful nurses. One time, I was laughing so loud at The Tonight Show that a nurse came to my room. I apologized for making so much noise. She told me that they were actually laughing at the nurses' station, just from hearing my laughter.

For twenty-three years I have been married to my great new husband, Harland. Together we have raised my son. We have laughed and loved. Harland has been beside me in every one of the challenges I have faced. He supported me in every way in my effort to earn a Master of Arts in Teaching, in French. I was able to travel and study in France. Even this wonderful time was not easy, however. We arrived in Paris on the 100th birthday of the Eiffel Tower. All my fellow students attended the gala event. I missed this and many other sites on our trip, because I had to sleep. Unspeakable fatigue was my travel companion.

**"Some family members have been repelled by my scars, embarrassed by my slow progress in the beginning, and even anxious about my mental stability. I know now that this was never about me. I had lost much, and people close to me feared they had also lost me. They were afraid I would never be the same. I am not."**

I can now laugh at many things that have happened. For example, I was counseled that I could earn my master's degree in only one year. It took me five years to complete.

Some family members have been repelled by my scars, embarrassed by my slow progress in the beginning, and even anxious about my mental stability. I know now that this was never about me. I had lost much, and people close to me feared they had also lost me. They were afraid I would never be the same. I am not.

Finally, I look back at this journey of twenty-seven years, and I am thankful. Every good thing that happens is like a gift. Every bad thing is merely a problem—one that I can find a way to solve. Sometimes I need help, and I ask for assistance. Sometimes I am very lonely and even angry. I find that friends, family, piano playing, reading, and knitting keep me happy. I had to find all of these treasures again in my life.

Back in May 1980, when I was in a coma, Mt. St. Helens exploded. I have no real memory of this event. And isn't memory strange? I have now seen numerous documentaries of this tragic eruption, and I feel like I do, in fact, remember it.

Like Mt. St. Helens, in 1980, my life exploded. I think, from the outside, one could see my life as one large trail of debris, much like the mountain. A closer look might show small, but real signs of new life. I think so.

❦ ❦

### Understand the changed brain.

It is important to understand the changed brain, especially when an injury is invisible. When the survivor looks good, people can mistakenly assume that all is well in the brain. Because all is not well, brain-injury survivors can feel sad, lonely, or isolated. Family and friends can help by understanding the limitations and challenges of the changed brain, including those that are hidden. For instance, short-term memory loss can affect learning, reading, and communication. Fatigue can be a ever-present challenge affecting all areas of life. Carepartners can assure those who have sustained a brain injury that they are loved and respected by recognizing the reality of the issues that brain-injury survivors face.

> ❧ "Recovery is a process. It can't be hurried, and it isn't a straight line up. Relax with the process and recognize that you need to look back at least six weeks to see your progress."
>
> STROKE THRIVER'S GROUP MEMBER

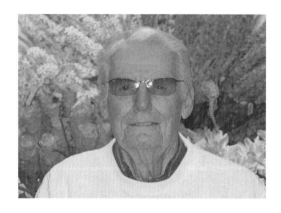

## I've Got to See Dr. Fixit

*by* Bill J.

There is an old proverb: "Wherever you go, there you are." That's very clearly true of the body, but not the mind—at least not my mind, the morning I had a stroke. A switch went off somewhere, and my brain would not respond to the signals I thought I was sending.

I was alone and totally confused. There was no pain; my only sensation was of a tiny bean inside a hollow gourd that, if tilted left or right, would rattle like a maraca.

Time meant nothing. I was going nowhere, and the only thing that was on my foggy screen was "I've got to see Dr. Fixit." This statement was all I could utter.

At some point I stood up, and it felt like my head kept rising, but my body remained fixed. This was a very strange feeling. Sitting again, my head returned to its normal location. Eerie!

My wife came in from errands, said hello, and I repeated my silly phrase, "I've got to see Dr. Fixit." She asked me if I was okay, and she got the same response. Then she phoned my daughter, and she too got the same answer, "I've got to see Dr. Fixit." They called 911, and very shortly a police officer came and gave me oxygen. Within minutes I was back to a semblance of normalcy. When the paramedics arrived, I was feeling much better and wondered, "Why all the equipment?" When they briefly removed my oxygen mask, I found out why. I slipped back into Never Never Land.

After the paramedics reattached my mask, I was again fairly lucid during the trip in the ambulance. What can you add to such a trip? In the ER I didn't observe any smiling faces, and I was beginning to wonder if I was looking at a grim scenario indeed.

The following day the pace quickened. Aside from tests on my body, I was now pushed from one floor to another to face myriad machines—some friendly, others rather fearsome. And the search went on. What caused the stroke, and where was its origin?

With a number of issues still unresolved, I was released. In a few days my wife noticed that I was having trouble with my speech. Back into the hospital I went, with a second stroke. I was given an angiogram, and the origin of the stroke was pinpointed.

The surgeon, who was going to operate, stopped by my bed and told me what happened. They located, up through the left carotid artery, an obstruction shaped like a shepherd's hook that had collected mushy plaque over time, then had let go and taken the blockage with it. The bent crook was an ideal place for the buildup of plaque.

The surgery was performed successfully, but later I was advised that I had a problem with my speech. It was strongly recommended that I take therapy. All I had to do was put some phrases together that made sense, and go from there, right? Wrong! It was the toughest job I've ever had to do. There was no reference point, because there was no meaning to a sentence. I was frustrated and felt: I may never get out of this mire.

When I took simple tasks home, it turned out to be a monumental endeavor to complete most. Matching words with their opposite meanings was a significant challenge, and I frequently asked my wife, "Does this look right?" It became an embarrassment to me when I couldn't respond to basic instructions from my therapist, but it was not for lack of trying.

**"Finally, a ray of hope broke through my brain desert, and logic took over with modest progress. At first, early on, time tests, writing tests, and memory tests, were a chore, due to my difficulty. Now they were proving to be a catalyst for faster improvement."**

Finally, a ray of hope broke through my brain desert, and logic took over with modest progress. At first, early on, time tests, writing tests, and memory tests were a chore, due to my difficulty. Now they were proving to be a catalyst for faster improvement. With short stories, quicker responses to questions, and memory answers, everything rapidly cleared, and I became fairly articulate—not a Rhodes Scholar quite yet, but able to say, "Good morning!"

In summation, I have high praise for the police officer and paramedics who got me to the hospital in under one hour, the fine surgeon who performed surgery and found the problem that caused the stroke, and the wonderful person who got my speech reoriented into a semblance of lucidity.

**Get the most you can out of rehab.**

There are a number of things that affect your progress during rehab. How much are you willing to practice? To re-learn skills, you will have to practice them many times. By repeating actions over and over you can build new neural pathways in your brain. It's a good idea to incorporate the things you love to do into your therapy. For instance, gardening is a great way to practice hand movements. Rehab is much easier when you have the support of your family and friends, whether they drive you to your appointments, practice with you, or simply cheer you on. But perhaps the most important thing is to bring to rehab your commitment to the process of recovery. You need to make an ongoing commitment to continue to try new things after you leave the therapy room. This will not only make a difference in recovering your skills, but also add greatly to your enjoyment of life.

Even if it's been years since your stroke, it can be helpful to check in with a therapist. Therapy interventions are continuously evolving, and a therapy refresher course might encourage growth in new areas of your life.

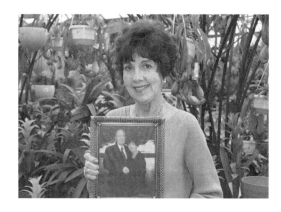

# A Real Overcomer

by Barbara

In February 1998, the damage report from Don's stroke looked ominous. Because of the extent and location of the stroke, the doctor didn't think that he would ever speak again. But as Don wrote sometime later, when he was journaling about his life, "I fooled them, and after eight months in speech therapy I was able to talk."

The road back to verbal communication was filled with all kinds of wonderful surprises, beginning just a few days after his stroke.

Surprise #1: He couldn't talk, but he could sing! I walked into his hospital room, and he was so excited. He was standing up, and all of a sudden he started singing "Jesus Loves Me." There wasn't a dry eye in the room as he repeated this performance for all who entered.

Surprise #2: When a person experiences challenges to their expression of speech, there is "speech therapy." Having had no need of such skills before, we didn't realize what miraculous changes in recovery of speech could be accomplished under the gifted direction of a speech therapist. Don's doctor had arranged for a very special woman who would be his chief cheerleader over the coming months, re-introducing him to the ability to talk.

Surprise #3: When God designed our bodies, He made them to heal themselves when given the right input. We had the joy of realizing that new pathways for speech were being formed in Don's brain, replacing the damaged tissue. With professional guidance, and with Don practicing his assigned homework of reading and speaking the words out loud, those new pathways developed.

Oh, what fun we had in the speech-therapy office. Don went from barely forming words to actually telling stories. In the process, there were a lot of jokes told back and forth, bringing much laughter. There were also times when tears of joy were shed, when a major goal in speaking was accomplished.

> "We had the joy of realizing that new pathways for speech were being formed in Don's brain, replacing the damaged tissue. With professional guidance and Don practicing his assigned homework of reading and speaking the words out loud, those new pathways developed."

Many years ago I bought name plaques for us and our two children that gave the meaning of our names. Don's name, as found in the Bible, means "Overcomer." It's from Revelation 2:7. Don was a true overcomer. He lived up to his name. He was 65 years old when he experienced the stroke, but he had a strong determination to get well, and it paid off.

Surprise #4: By May of 1998 he had made such great progress that he was named an honored "stroke survivor" at Fairview Southdale Hospital for that year, and he was their representative at the annual

Minnesota Twins' "Strike Out Stroke Day." What a great day that was for him! He, along with stroke survivors from other Twin Cities hospitals, were honored in a pre-game ceremony. His family and speech therapist were all there, cheering him on.

On this day he was given another plaque, titled "Perseverance." The inscription read: "In the confrontation between the stream and the rock, the stream always wins, not through strength but through persistence."

On October 26, 1998, Don wrote a letter to his speech therapist: "You have been a great help. You've given me self-confidence. Thank you very much. It has been a long, slow process, but you persisted. Starting with the very simple and gradually taking on the more complex words and sentences. Even more difficult was the problem of shifting from thought to thought and coming up with the several meanings of the words. Thank you for not giving up on me. You had faith in me and I in you. Thank you for giving me another chance to learn."

Don was a computer programmer and worked with systems design. By the end of 1998 he was back working on his computer, keeping our nonprofit public charity running smoothly. He didn't do new programming anymore because of the stroke's effect on reasoning, but he was fully able to run the business, do our taxes, drive his car, and expedite the sale of our condo in order to move out to a home by a lake, which we had always wanted. He thrived out at the lake and even designed an addition to our lake home.

I look back on this time and am so very thankful to God for the new people who supported us in prayer, for new friends made, for new experiences, for times when we laughed, and for the gifted, talented professionals whose guidance and friendship will be appreciated forever.

**Read aloud to an audience.**

Donald found the following story on the Internet. As a speech-therapy assignment he read it out loud, to the great delight of his neurologist and speech therapist.

> A priest was walking along the school corridor near the preschool wing when a group of little ones were trotting by, on the way to the cafeteria. One lad of about three or four stopped and looked at him in his clerical clothes and asked, "Why do you dress funny?" The man told the boy that he was a priest and that he wore the uniform priests wear. Then the boy pointed to the priest's plastic collar insert and asked, "Does it hurt? Do you have a boo-boo?" The priest was perplexed until he realized that, to the boy, the collar insert looked like a bandage. So the priest took it out to show him. On the back of the collar were raised letters giving the name of the manufacturer. The little guy felt the letters, and the priest asked, "Do you know what those words say?"
>
> "Yes I do," said the lad, who was not old enough to read. Peering intently at the letters, he said, "It says, 'Kills ticks and fleas up to six months.'"

Though reading out loud can be scary, it's an activity that speech therapists highly recommend, because it can help free you from anxiety and fear and give you the boost of confidence you need to work on your communication skills. That is the goal of speech therapy. It wasn't easy for Donald to read his story, but when he did, laughter, tears, and applause followed the successful completion of this monumental task.

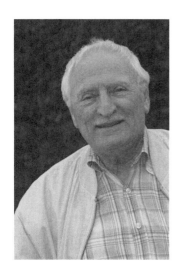

# Accepting What Is

*by* Bill R.

At the age of 77, I have just finished over two months of stroke therapy. Until recently, I had been lost to denial, not being aware that I had experienced a "mild" stroke. Now that I'm more fully acknowledging my new limitations, I have begun to accept that I must work around them. I know that denial is a great road when I feel overwhelmed, but I also know that it will only delay my recovery.

Things I have become aware of are: depression, frustration, anger, and resistance to the care that has been thrust upon me.

For me, complete recovery means the ability to drive again. This is the latchkey to the fulfillment of my expectations. It has been very difficult for the rehab staff taking care of me to establish a baseline and measure my progress. Some of the assigned tasks have been relatively easy, and others more demanding. I don't mean to offer resistance, but I have had difficulty accepting and redefining my new parameters. I am no longer so ambivalent about the whole episode. I feel my progress has been very good, and I will continue to work on some exercises to keep my mind clear and sharp.

My wife has made me aware of how much she loves and needs me, even though it has been a very trying and frustrating time for her. My wish is to see the time when her trust in me is restored, and I can reciprocate her kindness. I love her.

❧ ☙

**Denial slows recovery.**
After a brain injury, family members often say their loved one's personality has changed. The survivor may deny that any problems exist and appear to live with blinders on, unable to see and accept changes in function. Lack of recognition that your life has changed can slow the recovery progress. Families can encourage an individual to go to therapy, even when they may not fully comprehend the reasons for it.

## Rehabilitation Therapy

Therapy is a collaborative effort between physical, occupational, and speech therapies.

**Physical therapy** focuses on the large muscles of the body, both to improve strength, coordination, and balance and to restore motion. Physical therapists develop an exercise program to help survivors improve independence, and, if needed, they recommend equipment, such as walkers or canes, for balance and walking.

In **occupational therapy**, survivors work to regain arm and hand strength and coordination. They also address the typical activities of daily living, such as dressing and bathing. Skills such as paying bills, following a recipe to prepare a meal, making phone calls to set up appointments, and working on skills for driving are practiced as well.

**Speech-language pathologists** work to improve a survivor's ability to communicate with others, particularly those with aphasia, apraxia, or dysarthria.* **Speech therapists** teach techniques for improving memory, judgment, and problem-solving skills. Speech therapists also assess and treat various swallowing disorders and recommend a safe and appropriate diet.

Another type of resource person is a **physiatrist**, a medical doctor whose specialty is restoring maximum function lost through injury or disability. Physiatrists have completed training in physical medicine and rehabilitation and can prescribe medication. Their aim is to decrease pain and enhance function without surgery.

*See page 195 for a glossary of terms.

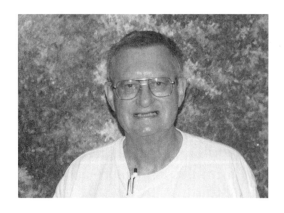

## Stroke Recovery Is a Marathon

*by* Jim

I was athletic, on a heart-healthy diet for 15 years, and a non-smoker, and still I had a major stroke on April 1 (no fooling). I had stroke symptoms again on November 14, after back surgery. I now take more golf strokes for 9 holes than I used to take for 18 holes. My new nickname is Reverend Strokes. Occasionally I laugh about my situation, because laughter is thought to be good medicine. So are movement therapy, deep breathing, and novel activities to stimulate growth of new pathways in the brain. They help to cope with deficits caused by permanent injury to part of the brain. But having a stroke is not an invitation to a pity party.

The day I had my stroke, I had just finished a 5K race, not knowing I was to begin a longer race (a marathon). I felt different. I tried to get into a car. It was the wrong car. Good friends found my car, put the key in the ignition (I could not do it myself), and invited me to a restaurant to celebrate finishing the race. I can still hear cars honking as I drove the wrong way on a one-way street. I remember thinking, "I have to get home and feed my dogs." Four days later I learned that I had had a massive stroke (the size of a handball), which changed my life forever. I lost names of people and places. I had to learn English a second time. My brain was changed.

**"Having a stroke is not an invitation to a pity party."**

There's hope after stroke. I'm a survivor. I am writing a book about cutting-edge research techniques to effect a speedy recovery from brain injury. I've attended stroke seminars at three different hospitals to gain insight into my stroke and available resources.

As an avid athlete, I believe three ingredients are necessary in ongoing recovery:

(1) Use it or lose it. Break things into small steps that are doable.

(2) Your brain is flexible but needs retraining. The brain can change itself. To begin an effective recovery, just start, like a marathon, one step at a time. Growing new pathways in the brain takes time and tenacity.

(3) Practice healthy nutrition. Eat a heart-healthy diet to nourish the brain with good circulation and vital ingredients.

**Rehab is ongoing.**

When you leave rehab therapy, your rehabilitation is just beginning. You are your own best therapist. As Jim discovered, the brain can form new pathways if you are willing to work hard and be tenacious. Sometimes a part of your brain that wasn't injured may take over certain activities that used to be controlled by the injured part. Jim demonstrates how proactive individuals, family members, and friends must be in seeking out resources that can improve performance. Challenging yourself to improve, one step at a time, every day, is the key to lifelong progress.

❧ "Trust your therapists."

STROKE THRIVER'S GROUP MEMBER

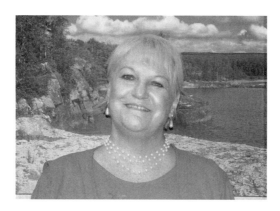

# I Have Graduated Out of First Grade, I Think

*by* Glo

I had a stroke two days after my heart surgery.
A speech therapist came into my room to test me.
I just wasn't sure what that entailed.

"Tests," I'd call them.
They reminded me of tests I had given students at school.
When I realized I couldn't pass them, I was completely devastated
    beyond anything I could comprehend.
I believed that I would be at a first-grade reading level the rest of
    my life.
What was happening to me?
Would I be able to learn again?
Would speech therapy help me understand why my brain was not
    working properly?

What was wrong with my brain?
Would I heal? I didn't know. I didn't know. I was worried.

I knew something was wrong with my brain.
I couldn't use my right hand to feed myself.
Terry came to visit me that night and saw that I couldn't hold a fork
    or a spoon. Later on he told me that he cried when he left my
    room that night. He had never seen me so helpless.
What was wrong with me? Would I be like this the rest of my life?
Who would take care of me?

I was assigned a speech therapist for six weeks.
I thought to myself, "Who are you?" and "Can my brain be fixed by
    you?"
So many questions. So many thoughts.
Can my brain be fixed by you?

I remember my therapist giving me tests to recall information.
I didn't do so well.
She'd switch to another test and have me memorize symbols that
    stood for words.
Then I was to read the words. I couldn't remember the words for the
    symbols.
I felt like a first grader reading letters (symbols) and not being able
    to understand the word.
I was a first grader. I was a first grader.
For once I understood their frustration.
I was one of them. No wonder school is difficult for some children.

I was one of them. I was.

Gradually, as our sessions passed, I "graduated" to doing creative writing assignments. I was assigned random words, and she'd tell me to write a story using those words.

Somehow . . . the randomness . . . or the creativity . . . helped me. I could take the words and create a story without stumbling.

I found the exercise exciting and so creative.

I was energized by the experience.

I was feeling not so first-grade-ish.

I continued my sessions and became more and more competent at writing.

I found the writing to be comforting and enhancing.

My confidence began to grow.

I began to see that there was a light at the end of the tunnel.

When I was a first grader, I hadn't imagined that there was an end to the tunnel.

Alleluia. There was.

As I grew with writing creatively, I grew within myself.

I grew believing that I could do better than I had done in the hospital when they had read me a story about Farmer Brown.

All I knew after they read me the story about Farmer Brown with 6 cows and 15 chickens is that . . .

Farmer Brown was just Farmer Brown . . .

Or was there even a Farmer Brown?

My brain needed healing. It needed healing.

Week after week, my writing exercises increased.

Exercise, exercise, exercise.

My brain needed exercise.

Thank goodness that my brain accepted the exercise.

I wasn't sure if it would.

I was amazed that it would stretch like a muscle or exercise band.

My mind really amazed me. I was so, so surprised.

It kept on working . . . and kept on helping me believe I would
     recover.


I'm not sure if this is the end of my story.

I just know from where I was (in the first grade)

And where I am now (fill in the blank) _____.

That I survived my stroke and became better.

I had never been through anything like this.

I felt like Magellan voyaging around the world.

Where will I land? What will I find?

Questions, questions, questions.

Magellan. Me. Magellan. Me.

The world. My recovery. The world. My recovery.


I learned that my therapists were my spirits, my forces, my coaches,
     my "you'll get through this" leaders who led me along the path
     through recovery from a stroke.

They became my paddle when I couldn't pull alongside the canoe.

They were my trainers when I couldn't lift that 12-pound bar over
     my head.

They were what I needed to become.

Therapy was what I needed at that point.

My therapists were my guides when I got lost.

They were my cooks when I forgot the basil.

They were my stepping-stones when I fumbled and fell down.

They saw in me hope and improvement, complimenting me and
    becoming my cheering section.

Without them, I did not see much hope.

**"My mind really amazed me. I was so, so surprised. It kept on working . . . and kept on helping me believe that I would recover."**

Therapy became an important part of my life—

A source of my confidence, my intelligence, my
    guidance, my drive, my ego.

I was raised from first grade to . . . soon to be a
    second grader?

Without them, I would not be the person I am
    today.

It amazed me that I had the ability to improve.

Without their confidence in me, I would still be in the first grade.


Thank you all, thank you, my friends.

I have graduated out of the first grade, I think.

Second grade doesn't look so hard now.


Soon to be second grader,


Glo

**Find creative ways to express yourself.**

Glo asks, "Can my brain be fixed by you?" She goes on to learn how hard her brain can work when guided by a speech therapist. Strategic and creative exercises can stimulate the adult brain. This, in combination with healing, can renew your confidence and enhance your recovery from a brain injury. While you exercise your brain, have a good time by trying something new. Glo is a retired schoolteacher who overflows with creative ideas. She tried her hand at poetry. You might write a poem or make up words to a song. The more you try, the more confident you will become.

ᕤ "Believe in yourself."

STROKE THRIVER'S GROUP MEMBER

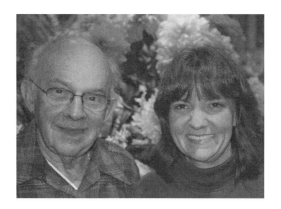

# What I Learned from My Stroke

*by* Harry and Barb

Things I have learned from the stroke:

- Have patience, healing is a slow process.

- Don't give up.

- Pay attention to directions from therapists. They are trying to help.

When I look back, I am surprised at what I had to re-learn—and did re-learn—such as eating with a fork, drinking from a glass, and tying shoes.

> Barb is Harry's daughter. Here she writes about how she learned to let go, as her father's therapy progressed and he became more independent.

After my dad's first stroke, he recuperated very quickly. After the second stroke, his right side was affected, and the doctor determined that he needed speech, occupational, and physical therapy. I was much more concerned after the second stroke because he was so much weaker. He also had some problems with memory, and I was worried that he would not fully recover. Since that time, two months ago, he has made tremendous progress. I believe that his positive attitude and his sense of humor have helped him to recover so quickly.

**"My initial instinct was to try to help him by doing everything I could for him. I gradually came to realize that this was not in his best interest—doing everything for him was comforting to me, but did not really help him."**

I have learned to step back and let him progress at his own pace. My initial instinct was to try to help him by doing everything I could for him. I gradually came to realize that this was not in his best interest—doing everything for him was comforting to me, but did not really help him. I have learned that I need to let him do things on his own and to help him only when he asks for it. I suppose I have learned to let him go, instead of trying to protect him, the same as he did for me as I was growing up.

## Learn to let go.

Barb's story illustrates what, for family members, can be one of the most challenging aspects of recovery. Because progress fluctuates daily, family members need guidance in knowing how best to help their loved one, without taking away independence. Rehab therapists teach family members how to help in positive ways to achieve the rehab goals.

## Use your whole body.

Survivors often focus their energy on strengthening the arm or leg not affected, preferring their stronger side for most tasks. A better approach is to use the weaker side as much as possible. For a fuller recovery, it's important to work the body as a whole and not favor one side over the other. Movement and repetition of tasks can help regain function in the weak, affected side.

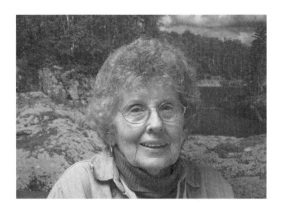

# Make a Difference

*by* Maria

Maria is a compassionate and caring presence at bedside. As a seasoned peer visitor, she mentors new peer visitors on the stroke unit. When Gary first started peer visiting, he was very nervous. But Maria's presence calmed him. As Gary says, "Maria is really dedicated. We help each other, fill in for each other. Sometimes I talk to a family member while she talks with the stroke survivor." Maria often shares a poem called "Strive & Conquer" with the families of stroke patients in the hospital. Gary's wife, also now a peer visitor, remembers Maria sharing the poem, written by another stroke survivor, and talking with her after Gary's stroke more than five years ago.

I had a stroke on March 20, 2001. It was a very terrible thing for me. I just can't talk. When I was in the hospital I saw the speech therapist twice a day. When I got home, after six days, we came three times a week. It was a very interesting time and it went fast.

After a stroke, we must learn to retrieve the names of objects and to put words together in sentences. I went to therapy for three months and then came back a year ago. I still have trouble with nouns and people's names.

When I was in the hospital, my husband brought in cards. We played cards all the time. I really loved bridge, and I started playing right away. My husband and children have helped me. I couldn't have done it without them.

I love being a peer visitor. I have been doing it for over five years. I work Mondays and one Saturday a month. I like visiting these people. Some of the families are very supportive. I encourage the person to talk, and they really open up to me.

Before I had a stroke, I didn't know anyone who'd had one. Just getting to talk to someone who knows was so important. Now, it feels so good to help. I feel so appreciated.

❧ ☙

**Peer visitors offer support to new stroke survivors.**
The peer visitor program has been an integral part of the Fairview Southdale Hospital Stroke Program for more than six years. This program began with seven carefully selected stroke survivors who went through extensive training. Sixteen volunteers now visit new stroke survivors. "It's a very frightening thing after a stroke. It's just scary, because you don't know what's going on. Until you've been there a day or two, it's just panic city," says Jim, a veteran peer visitor.

Some volunteers visit on the stroke unit. Others assist with classes and support groups or visit with survivors in outpatient rehab. Stroke peer visiting is also a vital part of other hospital stroke programs in our community.

Volunteer training has two parts. The first involves four sessions of StrokeWise, general-education classes open to any stroke survivor. The classes help the volunteers understand that every stroke is different and that families each cope in their own way. The second part of the training consists of five peer visitor classes, which include specific skills the volunteers will need, such as empathetic listening. "The peer-visitor training opened my eyes to other avenues of helping. It also changed the way I react in encounters with other stroke survivors," says Dennis, a new volunteer.

Both the selection process and the education are vital to a quality program. The StrokeWise classes and peer visitor training program are based on the American Stroke Association's peer visitor program kit (now called ShareGivers).

The program works smoothly on the stroke unit with cooperation between nurses and the volunteers, with visits taking place six days a week. Mary, a peer visitor for six years, says, "We may walk in on the patient's second day—not an easy time. I think our visits are meaningful to most, and there has always been a positive response."

Again and again, stroke patients who have recently left the hospital speak highly of the peer visitors. They may not remember the nurses or doctors, but they do remember the peer visitors. Professionals are able to discuss the facts and physiology of a stroke, but only stroke survivors can say, "I have been there, and there is hope for your future."

Maria shares this poem with new stroke survivors and their families.

### Strive & Conquer

Yesterday I was just like you
today I can't speak
and part of my body
quit working on me
they tell me I had a stroke
My mind still works
but I can't communicate
my hand and leg refuse to obey
It scares me to death
it makes me so mad
but I'm a fighter
and I won't take this lying down
My family is devastated
I can't comfort them with words
they feel they lost so much of me
but I'll come back
as far as God permits
So tell everyone to keep the faith
because I know you love me
and I love you, too
I'll strive, and I'll conquer.

DIANE HANNER, STROKE RECOVERY CENTER,
PALM SPRINGS, CALIFORNIA

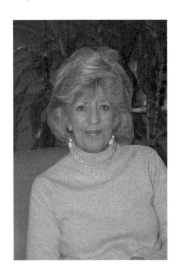

# The Mysterious Helper

*by* Sharon

As a task in speech therapy, Sharon, a stroke survivor, writes about her mother's experience with a generous stranger. Writing has helped Sharon organize sentences, express complex ideas, and use new vocabulary.

I'd like to share an extraordinary incident my mother experienced several years ago. At the age of 80, she was still very active, mowing her own yard, helping out at church, and taking care of the home she loved and had lived in for 45 years.

She went to the shopping center one day, like she had so many times over the years, and when she came out of the mall she couldn't find her car. After walking up and down the aisles, she was getting visibly upset. All of a sudden a man walked up behind her and asked if she needed help. He was dressed in a pilot's uniform and carrying a briefcase. She told him she couldn't find her car. He told her to get in his car, and they would drive around and find it. Instead of going into the shopping center and asking security for help, she went with the stranger. After several minutes of driving around, they found her car in a different parking lot, on the other side of the shopping center. She had entered through a different door, not the one she usually did.

If you had known my mother, you would know that you couldn't do anything to help her without her wanting to pay you back. This time was no exception. She tried to give the stranger money for his trouble, but he refused it. She asked him for a business card, which he gave her. It said he was a pilot for Northwest Airlines. She had him write his home address on the back of the card. When she got home, she wrote him a thank-you card for helping her and included the money he had refused to take.

A couple of weeks later, she received a letter in the mail and recognized the return address as being that of her pilot. When she opened it, the money fell out, and there was a note from his wife. She said she couldn't accept the money because it couldn't possibly have been her husband that helped my mother that day in the parking lot—her husband had passed away five years earlier.

❧ ☙

### Accept help.

Some good things that come into our lives are truly mystical. In times of trouble, such as after a stroke, there is frequently a silver lining. Often it's the people that come into our lives. It may be a friend who becomes closer and lends a special helping hand. Or it may be a stranger reaching out to you. It's important to learn to accept help. It can be challenging to allow others to help you when you're used to doing things on your own, but witnessing the generosity of strangers is a powerful way to keep your spirits up. The story of the mysterious pilot has touched not only Sharon's mother but her entire family and everyone who hears it.

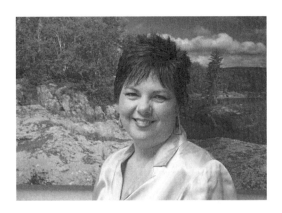

## No Direction Except Forward

*by* Val


My name is Val, and on July 12, 2005, at the young age of 45, I
had my first "event." I really hate the word *stroke*. *Event* suits me
better—maybe because it's like being at a party, and you are the only
one invited. There was no exact reason—nothing I did wrong, and
nothing I did right—it just happened. That is my first lesson that I
had to learn, and I try daily to remember it.

Even from the beginning, I cried (a ton). But I said, "I can do
life like this." However, you still have to find out *how* you are going
to do it. So, beyond going to speech, physical, and occupational
therapy, and even going to a massage therapist, I feel you have to try
to find what is going to work for you. I have learned to be my own
activist. Make sure you like and respect the doctors and therapists;
they are an integral part of your healing process. The speech and
occupational therapists at the hospital were my cheerleading

section, and sometimes I just needed their shoulders to cry on.

It has always been very difficult for me to roll with the punches. Prior to my event, I would just work harder to get the results needed. Now I work daily on rolling with the waves, because, unfortunately, some of the end results are truly out of my control. I'll start a word, and it will come out wrong. Sometimes I can change the word, and sometimes I can't, so sometimes I just make a joke out of it.

After my brain injury, my speed was definitely slower, but I was moving forward. About six months later, I began having seizures. My driver's license was put on hold. This was another definite setback. It is hard to be a realtor without a license. Unbelievably, my business partner, co-workers, friends, and especially family would drive me back and forth to work. They were truly there for me. I needed to put my pride aside and just appreciate all they did for me. I realized I really did have something to offer, and people would rather have a slower Val than no Val at all. I work a little slower and I am time sensitive, but it was important to get back to some normalcy. Find what will make you heal faster. I now know there will be no 100 percent, because I had this event that I need to deal with. One minute I can be clicking away, and the next I must lie down and take a break. My mind simply needs a rest for one to two hours; then I am ready for the next part of the day. This is another daily reminder: Listen to your body.

**"One minute you can be clicking away, and the next it is a must to lie down and take a break. My mind simply needs a rest for one to two hours; then I am ready for the next part of the day. This is another daily reminder: Listen to your body!"**

Here are some other things that have made my life easier:

- I carry a notepad all the time so I can always take short notes.

- Reading is still difficult for me. I now read short, positive stories that I can finish in one sitting.

- I park my car close to the same place all the time and, if need be, I jot the location down in my notebook.

- Writing is a constant reminder of what I have difficulty with. I keep it short. I type or have Wite-Out in every desk drawer.

- I exercise. All the doctors have said that because I was in good health when event #1 took place, that it made recovery a little better. Stay in good health.

- Sometimes it becomes very easy to let people do things for me. It's easier, less energy, less chance of failure. We really have to take the extra step to accomplish a goal.

- Keep track of your progress. I cannot keep up with a daily diary. Sometimes that works for people and sometimes it doesn't. I keep track by events—something that happened to me, such as my first written sentence, one-year anniversary, this story. Measure every little accomplishment and keep track of it.

I am learning it is okay to say the word *stroke*. It is important what comes next for me. Even a year and a half after my stroke, I am finding things that I need to attend to. I have started seeing a counselor, because I am angry and I feel I need to heal, deep down in my mind and in my heart. My life is no longer on autopilot. I am going to actually have to work at it.

**Rest is essential to the recovery process.**

Val is now working part time, but she finds her energy is quickly depleted. She wisely follows the lead of her body. Since she knows her brain needs rest, she takes a break every day to rejuvenate herself.

Feeling tired after stroke is extremely common. Sometimes this changes, but often it remains a fact of life after a brain injury. There are many reasons you might be feeling fatigue. Emotional changes, such as depression, anxiety, anger, sadness, and even boredom, can be a cause. Your brain may still be healing and working at neural reorganization. Rehabilitation is hard work for both your body and your brain. And on the other hand, if you aren't exercising, that can make you feel tired and cause you to lose muscle. Pain, weakness on one side, or increased spasticity in your muscles can wear you down. You may also be using your energy in different ways. Perhaps you now have to put forth your utmost effort to accomplish tasks that were easy before the stroke—even walking and talking may be challenging. Sleep could be harder to come by if it's disturbed by your brain injury, by worry, or by a lack of exercise and fresh air. Medications, illegal drugs, and alcohol can also affect the quality of sleep. For a list of ways to help you conserve your energy, see page 40.

## Seizures after Stroke

Stroke survivors sometimes experience seizures after brain injury. A major-motor grand mal seizure is a seizure in which consciousness is lost and the muscles of the body are forcibly contracted. Some people may mistake seizure symptoms for a stroke. You may jerk, your eyes may roll, and you may fall and pass out. Seizures may occur shortly after a stroke—or weeks or even months—after the event.

Seizures are not a disease but rather a response of the brain to adverse conditions, and are fairly common after a stroke. The normal electricity in the neurons builds up excessively until they excite adjacent neurons, and, in a chain reaction, all the cells discharge at once. This buildup of electricity in the brain causes the symptoms described above. Once the seizure concludes—and, usually, this happens spontaneously—the brain is exhausted, and the individual is left confused and quite drowsy.

Most seizures can be controlled with medication. Many medications are available, and a neurologist can work with you to find one with few side effects and hazards. If you have experienced a seizure, contact your doctor immediately.

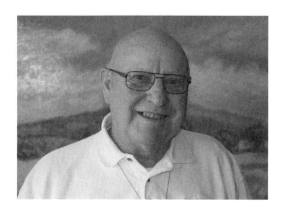

# Gone Fishing

*by* Bob

It was a bright sunny day. I was 69 years old at the time, fully retired for two years. My 83-year-old sister was up from Texas to spend some time with my wife and me. In the morning my sister and I had breakfast, and I left for the market. While shopping, I thought something was stuck to my right shoe. My foot seemed to be dragging. I checked my foot, and there was nothing there. With the shopping finished and at the check-out counter, I tried to write a check, but it was hardly legible. I drove home and mentioned what had happened to my sister. She insisted that I call my wife at work.

When my wife heard what had happened, she asked, "How do you feel?"

I said, "Just fine." About 20 minutes later, my wife, Mary, arrived home with a friend and neighbor, and 10 minutes later we were all at the emergency room. The staff did a bunch of tests. They kept me overnight. They told me I had a slight stroke, but all the tests showed everything was okay.

After being home awhile, I decided to take a nap while the girls played cards. I slept for an hour or so, and when I woke up I had lost the use of my right leg and arm. My face was a little droopy. Off to the hospital we went. The tests showed no cause for the stroke, just the damage it had done to the left side of my brain.

To recuperate and get back to where I was before the stroke, I started therapy. While in rehab with therapists Jen (occupational) and Shayla (physical), I decided there was too much fishing left to be done, and I was going to make this work. Jen said that after I could pick up coins with my fingers and put circles on wooden pegs, I could bring in my fishing rod and we would start casting a rubber plug. All the others in the room would have to duck to get out of the way. Shayla had me going up and down the stairs, going outside in the grass, up and over the curb, etc. We ended up making a fun time out of rehab. To help me with rehabilitation, I kept a basket by my favorite chair with a rubber-band gadget to strengthen my hand and weights and Therabands for my other muscles. During a ball game or movie, I could exercise without even thinking about it.

**"We ended up making a fun time out of rehab."**

Then Jen, the occupational therapist, sent me home with a list of things I could do. The list included playing the piano, washing windows and walls, doing the dishes, sorting buttons, kneading bread, and polishing silver. The next time I was at rehab I told Jen what a mess she had made for me at home. But I got no sympathy. Instead she said, "Bob, maybe we should do more tests on you. No one in their right mind would have shown the list to their wife." My wife, Mary, was so pleased with the list, she sent the therapists a thank-you card. She mentioned to them that I couldn't play the piano before my stroke or do most of the other things on that list.

※ ※

### Reduce stress to enhance your health.

Bob's ability to turn his rehab sessions into entertainment for himself and his therapists is an example of how he reduces stress in his life. By lowering his stress, he makes it easier for his body to heal.

Stress is your mind's reaction to anger, worry, frustration, or a feeling of pressure to perform or get things done. In response, your body releases hormones that make your heart beat faster, narrow certain arteries, and make your blood clot more easily. Lowering the stress hormones in your body is a powerful way to manage your risk factors and feel better. It's important to do something every day to manage stress by slowing your pulse, lowering your blood pressure, relaxing your muscles, and clearing your mind.

Here are some tips to reduce stress:

- Try to visualize positive outcomes to stressful situations, rather than worst-case scenarios.

- Seek out things that make you laugh—good friends, books, funny movies and TV shows.

- Avoid situations that are likely to increase your stress. If you hate grocery shopping, find a delivery service, or ask a friend to pick up your groceries.

- Exercise regularly. It burns up stress hormones and releases relaxing endorphins.

- Take care of yourself by eating healthy foods and limiting alcohol.

- Develop a support system. Share your worries. Ask for a ride or help with shopping and errands.

- Give yourself a treat. A massage, a movie, a hobby, or lunch with a friend can be great ways to relax.

- Pay attention to your breathing. Breathe with your stomach not just your chest.

- Breathe deeply.

- Listen to beautiful music. Relaxing instrumental music can activate alpha waves in your brain, which help induce sleep and relaxation.

- Meditate. Empty your mind of thoughts and worries by learning how to meditate. There are books, tapes, and teachers to help you learn this stress-busting technique. Or try Tai Chi exercise, often called "moving meditation." (See page 59.)

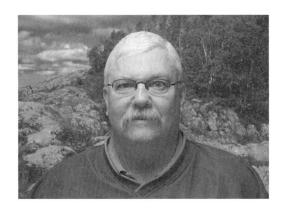

# Family Keeps You Going

*by* Gary

There are times when life really stinks. I look back on what my Mom said: "God never gives you more than you can handle." Well, Chris, my son, was born with an incurable disease. Suddenly, I was a single parent with two children. Chris was very handicapped. My brothers and I had just bought our parents' cabinet shop. Because of my brothers, I was able to raise Chris. I didn't have to put him in a home.

I met my new wife, Doreen. When I proposed, Doreen married me and my family. After Chris died, life turned to normal for a while. Then my brother, Lee, collapsed while the two of us were loading a truck, and he died instantly at age 46. That was another "stroke" of bad luck. Then I had a stroke. More than once I said, "You better lighten up, Lord—it's getting pretty heavy."

We are a very close family. Because of my visual defects and my brain being slow, I know what I'm trying to say, yet I panic sometimes. My brother and I decided he couldn't run the business alone, and we gave up our family business. I couldn't build. I couldn't read the numbers on the ruler for the specifications on cabinetry jobs. And I couldn't drive anymore.

Stick with your faith. I questioned why babies are put on this earth to die. Could it be that, through Chris, my faith has grown so much stronger? Chris always reached out and touched so many people. He held another hurting person's hand. I was blessed to have my son. Yes, you've got to have faith. Some day I'll know the answers to my questions.

**"I want to let other stroke survivors know that life isn't done. It's tough, but you've got to deal with what you've got. There's help. You can't just give up!"**

Why worry about things you have no control over? Pray about it. Good or bad, it will run its course. Don't get excited about materialistic things. If you're going to worry, find something really big to worry about.

Now I'm so excited. I've been in training for one year and am , a peer visitor, who volunteers to visit stroke patients in the hospital. I want to let other stroke survivors know that life isn't done. It's tough, but you've got to deal with what you've got. There's help. You can't just give up.

**Help a loved one with aphasia.**

As Gary said, he knows what he wants to say, but sometimes he can't get the words out. This problem is called "aphasia." Aphasia is a usually caused by an injury on the left side of the brain that limits the ability to speak, read, write, or understand what other people are saying. If the survivor in your life has aphasia, here are some things to remember:

- Include them in the conversation. Help them feel a part of things.

- Don't talk about the survivor as if he or she isn't there. Even if they can't respond, they can hear you and understand what you're saying.

- Don't correct their speech unless they ask you to.

- Encourage all efforts to communicate.

- Ask if they want help; don't just take over.

- Don't expect too much too soon.

- Don't promise they will recover completely. Recovery is a process and different for each person.

- Celebrate small improvements.

- Treat them as adults.

- If you don't understand something they said, ask them to say it again. Don't pretend to understand.

- Remember that people with aphasia tire easily. They may not be able to communicate as well when tired.

# The ABCs of Living with Communication Challenges

*by* the members of the Life in Bloom Aphasia Group

All things improve with time and hard work.

Believe in yourself. Things will get better.

Challenge yourself to do something different every day—
crosswords, sudoku, reading.

Daily "brain breaks" are important.

Each day, write down new ideas that occur to you.

Faith in yourself and your abilities.

Give yourself time each day for reviewing and planning
activities.

Help stroke thrivers by sharing ideas of mutual self-
improvement.

Investigate new ideas.

Join in—your fellow survivors understand.

Know that we are all different. We don't need to compare.

Learn to slow down.

Measure success in small steps.

Never count yourself out.

Overcome fear.

Peek into a bookstore, and read, read, read.

Quiet your body and mind. Try Tai Chi Chih.

Recite a poem.

Sing—it helps the words come.

Tell yourself positive things

Use any tool that may help. Try the dictionary.

Visit museums, libraries, concerts to stimulate your mind and
    spirit.

Worry less, think more. And write, write, write.

X-cellent attitudes.

Yes I can! Speak, write, gesture, draw, communicate.

Zero effort = zero gain. Zero in on speaking clearly and slowly.

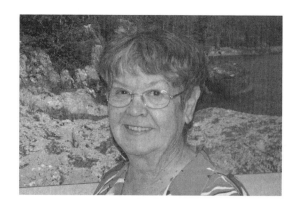

# Just Do It!

*by* Yvonne

Yvonne suffered a right-hemisphere stroke. When injury occurs on the right side of the brain, there can be challenges with concentration, vision, memory, problem solving, and reasoning. Organizing such mundane tasks as dressing and cooking can be challenging, since they involve completing steps in a sequence to achieve the desired outcome.

A therapist designed a task to help Yvonne with her focus and with her ability to put events in the right order. Yvonne was asked by the therapist to look up the following five words in the dictionary and use them in a story: *terrific, marvelous, ambition, appreciation, humorous.* Here is what Yvonne wrote:

This is a terrific day. The sun is shining with marvelous temps. My therapists are driving my ambition. Overall I have great appreciation for them. The message is always: Don't lose your sense of the humorous.

**Manage everyday life with simple tools.**

Yvonne keeps a pocket calendar and writes down one or two tasks to complete each day. "When I do a task, I say, 'It's done now, and I don't have to think about it anymore.'" Other simple tools that can help you manage day-to-day life after a brain injury include sticky notes and calendars. Taking regular naps can help rest your brain.

Achieving daily goals is challenging for a survivor who has suffered from a right-hemisphere stroke. It can be very easy to procrastinate. "I say to myself, 'Get up and do it! Get it done. Don't just think about it, because procrastination takes over your brain and gets you stuck,'" explains Yvonne. Successfully completing tasks has helped Yvonne improve her self-esteem and decrease her frustration.

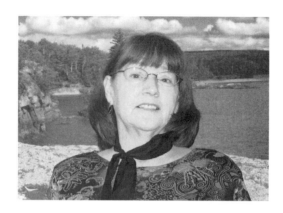

# Survival

*by* Sandy

Having a stroke is very devastating.
Sometimes you don't know who people are
even though you're aware that you should.
You'll often wonder why you aren't up to par.

Every single part of your body is affected.
Walking, reading, and writing are hard
because your eyes seem not to focus;
and walking means slipping, so you need a guard.

You'll have to go to therapy for a while
so you can be taught what you once knew.
The process can go slow or quickly.
The things you re-learn may be lots or a few.

Therapists will be patient and kind
helping and coaching you all the way.
Perhaps you'll find a new sense of self
and walk taller, feeling newer each day.

It has now been over two years since I experienced that harrowing climb up from the depths of a stroke. At the time, going through therapy, I felt I would never be independent again. Time was crawling, and complete recovery seemed unattainable. I fretted, I fumed. I denied I had a problem. Slowly, from my point of view— but quickly in my therapist's eyes—I did come back to almost full capacity. I have been told no one survives a stroke unscathed and I am no exception. However, most of the abilities I lost were able to be picked up and redefined by another section of my brain.

I will never forget the wonderful, caring, and understanding help of my occupational therapist and speech pathologist. They saw me through my hurt and confusion, and never faltered in helping me heal.

I feel I was truly blessed to be offered this new lease on life. Since the recovery phase, I have become a more confident person. Where fears hold me back, I'm learning to deal with them face forward. I have every intention of continuing my mental growth. I try to do crosswords, cryptoquips, logic puzzles, and jigsaw puzzles. I read thrillers, mysteries, espionage, and historic novels. I write poetry and stories. I like sewing and needlework. I meet friends for coffee regularly. I will fight as hard as I can to keep my brain from shutting down.

> "I feel I was truly blessed to be offered this new lease on life. Since the recovery phase, I have become a more confident person. Where fears hold me back, I'm learning to deal with them face forward."

I will be 59 years old this summer, and parts of me are showing and feeling the aches and pains of these years. Even so, I will continue to survive as long as I'm allowed that gift. And I will do so with humor, wit, and a large smile.

❧ ❧

**Your memory can improve with practice.**
Sandy describes a moment that many brain-injury survivors experience: "Sometimes you don't know who people are, even though you're aware that you should." Survivors often believe that they have lost certain memories. But many times, these memories are well preserved. What is actually affected is the ability to access the words to express the memories. Survivors learn to recognize that the memory is in the brain, they just need time to get it out. Like any skill, your memory for words gets better with practice. Here's a suggestion: Write down the names of things you find in your kitchen. Or write the names of people in your family on their photos. Labeling familiar objects and people can help trigger your memories.

## IMPROVING MEMORY

- Use all your senses. Make use of your eyes, ears, and sense of touch to remember things.

- Pay attention. Focus when someone tells you something.

- Tell yourself what you're doing as you're doing it. If you're going out for a few hours, as you close the door tell yourself, "I'm locking the door now. I'm putting the key in my pocket."

- Give yourself clear reminders. If you need dog food, put the empty bag by the door so you see it when you leave.

- Put things where you can't ignore them. If you need to return library books, put them in the middle of the table where you can't miss them.

- Keep things in the same place. This way, you won't have to wonder where you put your keys, remote control, or medicine.

- Chunk information. Instead of trying to remember each digit of a phone number, remember things in groups. For a number like 564-9876, think of 564 as one chunk, 98 as another, and 76 as a third.

- Use helpful tools. Use a calendar, daily planner, or sticky notes to remind yourself of what you need to do.

- Stay positive. People who feel good about themselves and the world remember things better.

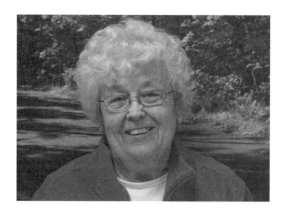

## Where Do We Go from Here?

*by* Roy E.

We're rapidly approaching the two-year anniversary of Shirley's stroke, which left her with what the doctors call aphasia. The stroke, a severe one, took away Shirley's four great loves: reading, bridge, cooking, and needlework.

We've learned that therapy—speech, occupational, and physical—does help, but both of us are a bit frustrated that improvement comes slowly.

We've also learned that I'm not a very good cook, and that Stouffer's is the best frozen entrée choice and man's best friend.

I've learned that I'm guilty of being an enabler, and I'm trying to back off and let Shirley make mistakes while trying to do things that are still difficult for her. Some progress here, but not enough. It is hard for me not to help too much.

Where do we go from here? We're going to attend a Minnesota Stroke Association program that starts soon—with an emphasis on speech therapy (which is Shirley's greatest need now). And we've also signed up for ongoing stroke-education classes. I know these things will help. I still keep hoping for a "magic bullet," a program or cure that will more quickly restore Shirley's great loves and talents.

Meanwhile, she remains the same lovely woman that I married some 55 years ago, and I still love her dearly.

❧ ☙

### Carepartners also need to care for themselves.

During the major changes that occur for the survivor after a brain injury, it's easy for spouses and carepartners to get lost in the shuffle. But carepartners are also at risk for depression. They often sacrifice their own physical and emotional needs to provide the best care for their loved one. This can result in (very normal) feelings of anger, sadness, isolation, exhaustion, and guilt. Carepartners need to pay attention to their own feelings and seek help when they need it. Support groups, physicians, counselors, family, and friends can help. See pages 196–198.

> ❧ "Carepartners need to try not to be too helpful and must allow survivors to do as much as they can."
>
> STROKE THRIVER'S GROUP MEMBER

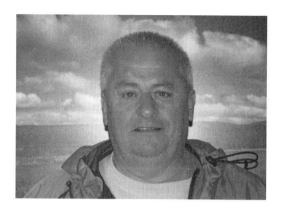

# He Scores!

## *by* Ron

Before my stroke, I didn't enjoy the journey I had to take to get to my destination. I just wanted to get there as fast as I could, sometimes stepping on people. I did not realize what an ill-mannered person I had become. Being too focused on a goal narrows your vision, and you don't see how it affects others. You end up going through life missing what's important between the start and the finish.

In a split second on July 9, 2004, all that changed. The stroke made me slow down. I now enjoy the smaller things in my day. I take time to observe the scenery. I look forward to what's around the next bend in the road.

My wife and I have always had that special feeling for each other. Words alone cannot describe the strength and complete love that is shown and felt. She's the best thing that has ever happened to me. She is the perfect partner, a tireless caregiver, and my motivator for thirty-six years.

Together we attacked our therapy with desire and fortitude, knowing that the road to recovery would be long and hard. Difficulty with comprehension and stamina had a grasp on my body and soul. The speech pathologists that worked with us were phenomenal. I told one of them afterwards that there were two people in my life I would never forget: "my drill sergeant from boot camp and you." We must remember that you can't sharpen a razor on velvet.

The biggest emphasis in therapy was put on homework—what we would do after the therapy sessions. Our recovery is ongoing and may never stop. Daily, we must go as far as we can, then go one step farther. If we fall, we have to get up. A failure can become a success, if we learn from it.

While waiting for a therapy session one day, I was reading an article in one of the medical journals. It explained the game of golf is a great way for stroke survivors to work on their recovery. After my wife read the article, we decided to take up the game. Along with our other methods of at-home therapy, this has become our favorite. Golf addresses my stroke challenges. To me, it's good exercise and fresh air. It makes me work very hard on controlling that emotional roller coaster. Anger management is tested, due to the frustration level that is a result of the game itself. It also challenges my memory. After each hole you have to count your shots for your scorecard. As bad as I golf, this can really be a test.

**"The stroke may have limited my activity, but it will never limit my spirit."**

Most importantly, golf gives us a relief from the stress and worry that goes along with recovery. Golf has become our new passion— and a family affair, with my sons included. We enjoy each other more than ever.

167

Out of every struggle comes some good. We have to look for the good. In the long run it will make us stronger. The stroke may have limited my activity, but it will never limit my spirit. The changes in my life have not been easy to accept. Change is hard for all of us. Wouldn't it be boring if everything stayed the same?

At this moment, I like where I'm heading in life and I am thankful to wake up for each new day. I see the whole experience as a blessing.

❧ ☙

**Exercise is good for both the body and the brain.**
After a stroke, you may think that exercise is the last thing you want to do, but a lack of physical activity can result in osteoporosis, joint problems, weak muscles, falls, cardiovascular problems, and depression. Your risk for another stroke is also much higher if you don't exercise. The guidelines from the American Stroke Association recommend 20 to 30 minutes a day of moderate aerobic exercise—that is, exercise that gets your heart rate up. The ASA guidelines say you can exercise in 10-minute bursts of activity two or three times a day with the same benefits. Try to do this at least three days a week. But talk to your therapist or doctor before you start any new exercise routine.

## EXERCISE AND HEALTH

Regular exercise reduces your risk for another stroke and promotes

- healthy weight

- better sleep

- more energy

- less anxiety, stress, and depression

- greater self-esteem

- healthier muscles, bones, and joints

- better range of motion and blood flow

- greater use of arms and legs that were weakened by the stroke

- stronger muscles, which can help you compensate if you have lost some function in your body

**"Treasure your time with family and friends."**

STROKE THRIVER'S GROUP MEMBER

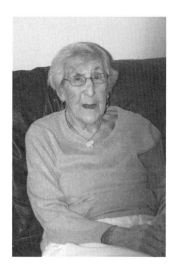

# A Second Stroke, a Smooth Sail

*by* Rae

When I get out of rehab tomorrow, I'll be singing praises for a second successful stroke battle. I had my first stroke in 2002, and I was totally overwhelmed by it. At 86, I had my second stroke, and I seem to have sailed through it. I am looking forward to a complete recovery.

**"My words of wisdom: Hang in there. Don't give yourself a chance to go over the 'Why me?'"**

I couldn't have been more surprised when the second stroke happened. I had dinner, sat on the sofa, and couldn't move. That's all I remember. When I didn't respond to a friend's e-mail sent the night before, she immediately came over and found me half on the sofa and half on the floor. She called 911, and I was swept away to the hospital. Since I'm a stroke peer visitor, I anticipated that another peer visitor would come to see me. I was glad to see the volunteer, because he knew my predicament.

I have volunteered at the hospitality desk at the hospital since 1987. I took classes to become a peer visitor when I was 86 years old. People have been amazing, their kindness and goodness. My care has been excellent. I didn't have time to bask in self pity. My words of wisdom: Hang in there. Don't give yourself a chance to go over the "Why me?"

❧ ☙

**Don't spend time on things you can't change.**
As Rae so wisely stated, "Don't give yourself the chance to go over the "Why me?" Instead of dwelling on the things you can't change, focus on those things you can and have done. To keep her focus on the positive, Rae is always pursuing new adventures, new ideas, and new friends. What can you do to keep from dwelling on the things you can't change? How can you celebrate your milestones?

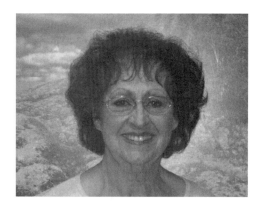

# Serving In Gentle Ways

### *by* Geraldine

Geraldine is a gospel singer who, prior to her stroke, regularly entertained residents in nursing homes. During speech therapy, she rediscovered her ability to vocalize by lifting and projecting her voice into a tape recorder. The two writing assignments below focus on the rewards she gained through her volunteer experiences before her stroke.

One day as I was visiting my grandma in the nursing home, I walked down the hall, greeting the people as I passed their rooms. There was a lady who was crying very loud, and there was a nurse with her. I visited with Grandma a few minutes, and the lady was still crying. I told Grandma I'd be back in a few minutes.

I walked into the lady's room. The nurse had left. I sat down next to her and put my arm around her and began to sing "Jesus Loves Me,

This I Know." After one time through, I asked her to sing with me, which she did. I asked her if she believed the words she sang. She said yes. I prayed with her, and she was quiet. I said, "I'll see you later," and left. Grandma was happy she stopped crying. The nurse wondered what I had done. I said I sang "Jesus Loves Me" and prayed with her. When I left the nursing home I walked by her room. She was quiet ,and I said, "Remember, Jesus loves you and so do I."

On a Sunday morning, I was playing the piano for a Sunday morning church service at the nursing home. The people were coming in and getting seated. I looked up, and in the first row sat a lady who looked familiar to me. As I looked at her, I thought she looked just like Mrs. Berry, one of my elementary school teachers. I thought, "Could it be?" The service began, and I sang a medley: "I Come to the Garden," "Just a Closer Walk with Thee," and "What a Friend We Have in Jesus." After the service, I could hardly wait to talk to the woman. She smiled and said, "Hello, Geraldine." She remembered my name even though 60 years had passed! That was a joyous reunion.

I volunteered at this nursing home for eight years and had many happy times there.

❧ ❧

**Use whatever helps you.**
You have the best resources for healing within yourself. Think about your past interests, and also those things you've always wanted to do. You might try signing up for therapy, asking for help, attending church, taking a class, or volunteering like Geraldine. Interacting with others improves skills.

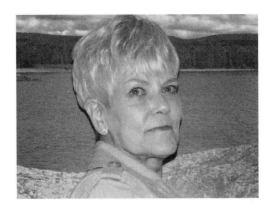

# I'm a Fighter

*by* Danette

I was a fighter from birth. I was born in a Catholic hospital in Grand Forks, North Dakota. The hospital was run by nuns. I weighed 3 lb. 2 oz. when I was born, and, until an incubator arrived, a nun kept me warm in her habit.

In 1986 my mother entered a nursing home, which was very difficult, following the amputation of her leg and a stroke. It was a roller coaster. As she was dying, I held her hands. I was sad but felt no fear. We strive and struggle. If I could wave a magic wand, I would want God to take us at the right time—just to take the pain away.

As a stroke thriver, I feel like I am on borrowed time here on earth, and I want to do everything I can while I'm here to help others. In my volunteer job as a stroke peer visitor, I visit new stroke survivors in the hospital to encourage them, but I also sometimes visit with those who are not going to survive. I learned from Mom that you must accept what happens in the dying process. Death and grief have been companions throughout my lifetime. It has made me a stronger person. I can take the hand of a person who is dying and hold it.

Life's a challenge. My motto is: "You have to get up." Your days are all different—some good days and some bad days—and you must accept what is dished out to you. Life goes on. I'm fortunate I can say, "I'm a survivor."

**"Life's a challenge. My motto is 'You have to get up!'"**

☙ ❧

**Know the warning signs of stroke.**
Know all the warning signs of stroke (see page 203), as the symptoms can vary from stroke to stroke, even for the same person. The sooner you can get to the emergency room of a Primary Stroke Center, the better. Minutes matter, so be sure that both you and your carepartners are alert to any problems. Call 911 if you experience any warning signs. It is also important to carry with you such information as your diagnosis, medications, and family contacts and phone numbers.

## CONTROLLING YOUR RISK FACTORS

Stroke survivors often express the fear of having a second stroke and, in fact, survivors of stroke do have a greater risk of stroke than does the general population. However, you may be able to prevent a second stroke if you can control the risk factors that contributed to your first stroke.

You must first know what type of stroke you had and why you had it. Was your stroke caused by a blockage in a blood vessel supplying the brain (referred to as an **ischemic stroke**), or by a ruptured vessel that bled into the brain (referred to as a **hemorrhagic stroke**)? Whether the stroke was hemorrhagic or ischemic, controlling your personal risk factors can reduce your risk of having another stroke. Focus on the things that you can change. It's important to take a close look at each risk factor with your healthcare provider and follow through with all the recommendations they suggest for management. Potential risk factors include high blood pressure, smoking, diabetes, high cholesterol, physical inactivity, and obesity.

Work closely with your doctor. Ask your doctor which medications are right for you. Anti-platelet agents, including aspirin, Aggrenox, and Plavix, have been used successfully for stroke management. Do not stop taking any medication without first talking with your doctor. If your stroke was caused by atrial fibrillation or carotid artery disease, you should discuss the medical and surgical treatment options with your doctor.

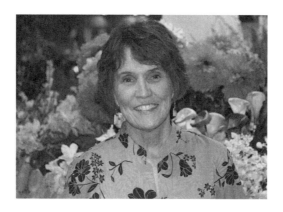

# The Present

*by* Margie

"My present, I need my present." My daughter, Liz, looked back at me quizzically, wondering what I was talking about. Liz was trying to get me out to the car as rapidly as she could.

The nurse on the Help Line had told her to get me to the hospital as quickly as possible. "Your mom is having a stroke."

"You want your present?" Liz pondered the words, and within a few seconds she said, "Your book, that's what you mean. That book you were reading all day yesterday."

I nodded in response.

The next eight or so hours were spent in the emergency room. Late in the afternoon, I was transferred to a room in the hospital.

That evening I encouraged Liz to attend her high school reunion. Liz left my book and my glasses on the table next to me. I thought reading would help me relax. I looked forward to returning to the novel I had been enjoying the day before. I opened to the marker and tried to focus on the page. The symbols on the page made no sense to me. It was as if I had become one of the learning-disabled students I had taught for the past 30 years. I tried for a minute or so to see if things improved, but when they didn't, I closed the book. Interestingly, I felt no sense of panic. "I don't seem to be able to read," I thought. "I'll have to think about that later." This rather blasé attitude had been with me since early that morning, when Liz was told I was having a stroke. I felt something like, "This can't really be happening to me, so I won't concern myself until the real verdict is in."

On waking the next morning, Sunday, I pondered the name of the hospital I was in . . . not a clue. I moved on to trying to think of the name of the city where my other daughter, Claire, lived. I decided that was enough thinking for the moment and returned to the "not much of anything going on" status of my brain.

Later that morning, I started to see many different therapists. This was both exhausting and rather overwhelming. I remember the last therapist of the day as "Ms. Speech." She tried a variety of things, including telling me a story about an older woman who lived in the country, and her son wanted her to move to town. However, when asked a series of questions about the story, I couldn't answer most of them. It was challenging to keep the content of the story in any sort of logical order. Everything I heard seemed quite confusing.

Monday dawned, and I went through my short morning quiz. Did I know the hospital I was in? The answer was still no. The city where Claire lived? Suddenly the word "Portland" arrived. This seemed like a major scientific breakthrough: 48 hours after my stroke, and I now knew where one of my children lived.

On Tuesday I woke to the devastating news about New Orleans after Hurricane Katrina, and my own, new-found awareness of the hospital I was in. After 72 hours, I now could articulate where I had been since Saturday. This wisdom is apparently a significant milestone on the recovery scale, because after another morning in therapy, the doctor discussed my release from the hospital with Liz and me. The suggestion was that I go to some rehab facility, but Liz had worked out a plan for home-based therapy. Late Tuesday I went home. That night I slept in my own bed.

On Wednesday morning, I knew where I was. It was amazing what a difference a day at home made. It was definitely easier to articulate my thoughts in a familiar setting. Liz and I started to map out the plans for the rest of the week: when therapists would come, when the visiting nurses would come, when a teacher would come to get my lesson plans for the first days of school. I had been working all summer to prepare for some new classes I was going to teach. Fortunately, I had set up some course maps, as it was hard for me to describe my plans in much detail. Even now, it is still difficult for me to explain things in proper sequence.

It was late on Wednesday, a day after I came home, when a great wave of anxiety descended upon me. I was no longer watching what was taking place from a safe distance. How would all of this turn out? Would I really be able to read and write again? Would I ever be able to talk fast enough so that I, to say nothing of my listeners, would still remember what I was talking about by the time I got to the end of the sentence? I did not sleep well that night.

It occurs to me now that I counted each day from the day of my stroke, like you do each day, for example, after the birth of a child. First you say, my child is 6 days old, but soon you start counting in weeks, then months. Eventually, time flows again, and the minute-by-minute accounting of what has happened becomes less important. After about six weeks of speech and occupational therapy at home, I graduated to the status of out-patient at the hospital three or four times a week.

I didn't always understand why my therapists asked me to do certain things. I stubbornly insisted to my occupational therapist that I didn't need to practice preparing a three-course meal, because I rarely cooked for myself. Now, any time I try to prepare a meal that involves anything more than placing something in the microwave, I think of my therapist. Thanksgiving dinner preparation is truly a nightmare, with too many dishes and a whopping headache that appears when I have to pay attention to more than one thing.

My speech therapist must have recognized that I felt pretty smug about my vocabulary output when I started working with her, but she was very cagey in using a variety of strategies to help push me forward. Sometime in November, I heard the story I had listened to when I was in the hospital—the one about the older woman who lived on a farm, and her son, who wanted her to move to town. This time I was able to answer all the questions. I wondered why it had been so difficult the first time. Experiences like this helped me realize how much healing my brain had done in the last three months with the help and support of many people.

With my therapists, I started to plan for my return to work. We focused a great deal on multi-tasking. As a high school English teacher who worked primarily with students who were struggling readers, I had to be able to juggle many balls at once.

I returned to school in January, hoping to make it at least until the end of the school year. I found I had to script all my lessons—words and ideas didn't flow naturally. My anxiety about losing my direction midway through a lesson became a reality. Simply put, my brain just didn't work as it had before my stroke.

As I looked at the disarray on my desk after the first three classes of the day, I felt like this was the manifestation of how my brain was functioning. I felt overwhelmed, trying to sort things out and prepare myself for the next two classes. After school, I needed a lot of time to regroup and then script the next day's lessons. I often worked until after 7:00 p.m., then headed home to sleep before it all started again.

**"A year and a half after my stroke, I find myself living quite a different life than I was before, but a life that is filled with many gifts— gifts like having the time to pay attention to my own health, time to volunteer, time to enjoy a walk around the lake, or, perhaps best of all, just having time to to think."**

Although I felt thoroughly overwhelmed, everyone kept saying how great I was doing. Part of this has to do with teachers being an affirming bunch, but also with the fact that I had no visible effects from my stroke. No one could see the brain turmoil I felt each day from simply trying to stay on top of the daily expectations of my work. Yes, I had been teaching for a long time, but never with a head so full of chaos. In March when the principal talked with me about a new schedule of classes she wanted me to teach the following school year, I knew I had to tell her I couldn't do it. She didn't believe me—but as soon as I said the word "retirement," I knew that was what I needed to do.

Though I don't miss working so hard, I really miss the kids at school, so I tutor students individually and find this not only manageable, but also very enjoyable. Just like cooking dinner, if I just have to prepare one dish, like the green beans, I do quite well.

A year and a half after my stroke, I find myself living quite a different life than I was before, but a life that is filled with many gifts—gifts like having the time to pay attention to my own health, time to volunteer, time to enjoy a walk around the lake, or, perhaps best of all, just having time to think. I feel like that "present" I wanted my daughter to bring with me to the hospital has become much more than just that book I was reading. It's this new life I'm living, which involves reinventing myself, but comes with the pleasurable anticipation of each new day.

## Be honest with yourself and others.

Your life will change after a brain injury. When your brain is injured, your abilities change in ways that are often invisible to others. Challenges in cognition, or thinking, can affect skills in organization, planning, problem solving, and memory. Frequently, these abilities aren't tested until you dive back into your daily responsibilities. Then you or your family may notice the extraordinary effort required to do things that came more easily to you before your stroke. Consulting with a neurologist or a neuropsychologist (a psychologist with a specialty in the relationship between the brain and behavior) can help identify exactly what has changed. Consulting with a rehab therapist can help you identify strategies for coping with these changes. Sometimes, this simply involves changing how you do certain tasks or jobs.

Some days will be easier than others. It's important that you be honest with yourself and your carepartners about your feelings, needs, and challenges. Margie had to admit to herself and her boss that it was time to retire from her job. She chose to use the moment as an opportunity to reinvent herself, by focusing on her strengths, as she looked to the future.

꙳ "I'm still in a book club, but I use books on tape."
STROKE THRIVER'S GROUP MEMBER

# Sharing His Gifts

## Charlie's Story

Before his stroke, Charlie had the ability to recall tiny details about the lives of people he met. According to his wife, Betty, if you told Charlie that his grandma had a hangnail 17 years ago, he would recall it. Losing some of his memory skills after the stroke was a big frustration to him. But it wasn't just tremendous memory skills that made people so comfortable with him. When Charlie listened to you, he really listened. He really cared about you. His attention was truly a gift. And he didn't lose that ability.

When his rehab therapists were asked to describe Charlie, they used words such as kind, warm-hearted, gentle, great listener, compassionate, and friendly. These positive aspects of his personality made him good at his job and successful in the important relationships in his life, including two highly valued stepsons. Despite his many losses with stroke and multiple sclerosis, he retained these many gifts.

Charlie never wanted anyone to know that he was sick. He dealt with many frustrations and losses, big and small. His wife recalled how the blind spot in his right field of vision allowed her to hide sometimes, unintentionally. He didn't find it as amusing as she did. Charlie used to be hugely dedicated to running and physical workouts, before physical changes from multiple sclerosis and stroke made it too taxing.

The rehab staff who knew Charlie and his wife and carepartner, Betty, expressed great admiration for their solid marriage. Betty showed such patience and understanding while coping with the hospital stays, the ups and downs, and the frustrations, along with her own physical challenges in recent years. Charlie showed his appreciation of her over and over again. The two of them liked each other's company and were truly a partnership. They shared humor and they dealt with many obstacles with both grace and love.

When he passed away in 2005, he was in training to become a stroke peer visitor. Hospital staff recognized his skill at listening and his ability to make people feel comfortable, both valuable assets to the program.

**"Charlie took the risk and traveled from fear to freedom. He was truly a 'stroke thriver,' not just a survivor."**

According to Betty, Charlie was initially reluctant to get involved at the hospital. Like many new stroke survivors, he was learning to cope and focused on what he could no longer do. But he appeared to recognize that others needed him. One of the new friends he made in peer-visitor classes recalled their first meeting, months earlier, when both were waiting for rehab appointments. She said, "Charlie was the first fellow stroke survivor who connected with me." She was so grateful he reached out to her when she was feeling very alone. "I'm so glad I told him how much that meant to me," she added.

Charlie taught those who came into contact with him about courage, perseverance, flexibility, patience, hard work, and the power of love and possibilities. In the words of his rehab specialist, "Charlie took the risk and traveled from fear to freedom. He was truly a 'stroke thriver,' not just a survivor."

**Turn fear into freedom.**

After a brain injury, it can take a great deal of courage to decide to step outside of your comfort zone. Sometimes fear is the only thing that holds you back from seeing how wonderful your new life can be with your changed brain. Using your strengths and gifts, re-learning skills you've known, trying new things, and putting yourself in new social situations are all ways to turn fear into freedom. Try thinking of the changes you've experienced not as deficits, but as challenges. What can you do or practice today that will help you turn fear into freedom?

❧ **"Welcome new experiences."**

STROKE THRIVER'S GROUP MEMBER

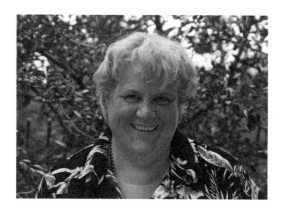

# It Can Be Done

*by* Lisa

You never know how quickly your life can change. I had a massive stroke on the right side of my brain, which affected my left side. My doctor called me with the news, and, to be honest, I did not believe him. I had a picture in my mind of a person who'd had a stroke, and I did not see myself in that picture.

I asked, "How am I going to live on my own? How am I going to work? What is going to happen to me?" It was as if I had walked into a brick wall. My sister, Christine, was with me when I received the news, and, like any older sister would, she took charge. She alerted my family. She had family members scheduled to be with me from that day through the summer months. I felt like she was the general in charge, and I was in the service. And that felt safe for me.

The effects of a stroke are very personalized—everyone is different. At first I had a difficult time tying my shoes or picking grapes out of a bowl with my left hand. During therapy sessions the therapist would put an everyday object in my left hand and ask if I knew what that object was. For the longest time, I was not able to determine what it was. When they put it in my right hand, I knew immediately what it was.

I had a real issue with getting from point A to point B. For example, if I wanted to move from the chair to the couch that was directly in front of me, I would walk the entire perimeter of the room. My sister would ask, "Lisa, why are you doing that?"

"Idiot," I'd say, "I'm going to sit on the couch." It made complete sense to me. Then Christine asked, "But why are you walking from the chair, around the entire edge of the room, and then to the couch?" Then she showed me exactly what I was doing. I had no idea I was doing that. I guess I needed to make sure a chair was really there, since my vision had changed.

I had lost my vision to the left in both eyes. I cannot see to the left unless I turn my head to the left. I did not realize, until I lost part of my vision, how important peripheral vision is. Because of my vision loss, I am not able to drive, which has really made a big change in my life.

Christine's daughter, whose education specialized in visual impairments, showed my family what my world now looked like. She brought eyeglasses for them to try on, with half of each lens covered. This blocked the view to the left for each eye. It's difficult to explain and hard to understand.

Friends I hadn't seen for a long time would ask me, "Can you watch TV?" I'd say, "Are you asking do I have one, or if I have cable?"

I can see to the left when I turn my head. But I usually choose to carry a white cane when I am out and about in unfamiliar areas. It keeps me safer by alerting others that I have a visual impairment. Also, I don't want anyone to think I just had lunch at Sally's Bar and Grill when I walk into a wall.

I spent several weeks at vision rehab, and I did learn how to work with my limitations. I learned new tips on how to read again. I had found myself skipping lines, and even whole pages. I remember reading cards sent by friends after my stroke. I'd say to my sister, "What's wrong with her? This doesn't make any sense." Christine would say, "Look to the left. There's a note, Lisa." Now I use a finger to follow the line on the page. I feel a little self-conscious at times, but it helps me with my reading.

I can still hear the voices of my sister and my therapist saying, "Turn your head, Lisa" or "Turn to the left." My vision-therapist's voice was always gentle. My sister, on the other hand, would yell it out, because she was family: "TURN YOUR HEAD! LISA, LOOK TO THE LEFT!" Now I can laugh about it, but there were moments, I can tell you, that I wanted to yell back.

It is difficult for me, at times, to realize that I cannot see to the left. For several months my family would tell people things like, "Lisa's not rude, she just can't see you on the left." I also was reminded of the fact that I had a vision limitation when I walked into a parked vehicle on the sidewalk—of course it was to my left. My friend was with me and was so concerned that I had hurt myself. At first I started to laugh, and then I said, "What the heck? Why is this truck parked on the sidewalk?"

I also spent time in speech therapy. I did not believe I had trouble with my speech, but I went anyway. My mom said, "Lisa, be sure and talk to your therapist about your lisp. I've always thought you had a little lisp."

I said, "Now you're telling me, after 46 years, that you've thought I have a lisp? Mom, I've got other things to worry about!"

When I first met my therapist, I introduced myself and then said, "Mississippi. M-i-s-s-i-s-s-i-p-p-i."

"Why are you spelling Mississippi?" my therapist asked.

"Since I am at speech therapy, I thought that would be a word you would want me to say and spell. I wanted to show you that I could do that."

She smiled and explained to me that there was more to speech therapy than just speaking. She spent some time working with me on the cognitive parts of my brain, and I realized I was having some difficulty.

I spent some time with a physical therapist, and that was often humorous. He would ask me to sit on this very large ball and balance, which I did for a moment. Then I would fall off the back of the ball. I would have to walk up steps, balance on one foot or the other, and do a variety of exercises. As with my other therapies, I had a great time and I laughed a lot.

There were some people who said I would never be able to return to work again. A person should never say *never* to Lisa. That gave me even more motivation to return to work. In fact, I was back to work full time a little over five months after my stroke.

My employers at the University of Minnesota helped me with some specialized services, such as a large-screen computer at my home and allow me the flexibility to do some work at home. The

challenge is my disabilities are hidden, but the white cane helps.
I also have fun with it at the new-student orientation meetings
I conduct. They assume I have no vision, so when my co-worker
points out someone with a question, I'll say something specific like,
"Oh, you mean that woman in the yellow shirt?"

Once I returned to work after my stroke, I felt
I was the office expert in regard to disability issues.
Many of the staff would come to me with questions.
I do feel I can be an educator about stroke, and I
am probably a better employee now. I concentrate
harder because I don't want to mess up.

What I found out during this journey, which
I continue to be on, is that laughing and humor
are critical components in getting healthier. Your
attitude has a lot to do with how you will progress.
Once I realized that I'd had a stroke and that
my life would be different, I was determined to
make everything work out. I had to look at things
differently. I had to realize that I was still able to
live an independent life, but I may have to make
some changes in how I did things. I was not willing to stop living.
I would not allow the fact that I could not see to the left, unless I
turned my head, be an obstacle for me.

I believe I have two birthdays: my actual day of birth and the
day I had my stroke. By all accounts I should have been in a coma on
April 21, but I wasn't, and that is something to celebrate. So every
April 21, I celebrate my life and how lucky I am to be alive. My first-
year anniversary of my stroke was over the Easter holiday. I wanted

> "Once I realized I had a stroke and that my life would be different, I was determined to make everything work out. I had to look at things differently. I had to realize that I was still able to live an independent life, but I may have to make some changes in how I did things. I was not willing to stop living."

to be with my family in Michigan, so I flew home for the weekend. I told my family, "All I want to do is drive a car."

After Easter services, the church parking lot was completely empty. My nephew pulled up with his car, and he was dressed in protective gear—driving glasses, gloves, and a helmet. He said, "Aunt Lisa, get in the car, and let's go."

I drove around the parking lot honking the horn, pulling into parking spots, backing up. You would have thought there was a parade in town. My family was standing on the side lines, cheering me on. Of course, as I drove by them, they would back up. I had a theme for this Easter event: "Christ has Risen, Lisa has driven."

Living with a stroke is not easy, but it can be done. I thank my family and friends for sticking with me. As I am reminded every single day, when I get up in the morning, I am still in the game.

❧ ☙

**Don't drive after a brain injury until you know it's safe.**
It may not be safe for you to drive after you've had a brain injury. You may not react as quickly as before your stroke. Medications, visual changes, weakness, or fatigue can distract you or limit your ability to drive safely. You may find it challenging to turn your head or body to check blind spots. Changes in judgment, memory, or perception, can negatively affect your driving. Even if you feel that you're ready to drive, you should get a complete evaluation to be sure. Ask your doctor and care team to tell you when it will be safe for you to drive again. Holding off on driving may feel like a personal loss, but it is also an issue of personal responsibility. You don't want to put yourself and others at risk.

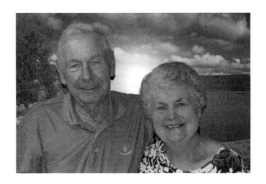

# Recipe for Romance

*by* Jack and Barb

It's a marriage made in heaven—48 years together, and Jack and Barb have faced many challenges, including Jack's four strokes. But instead of letting the difficulties they've had to face get in the way of their love for each other, this couple has remained strong. Though Jack is different today than he was before the strokes, Barb's appreciation for the man he is now grows every day. "The gifts that unfold as you live and grow together are surprising," Barb says. The couple give their advice for keeping love and romance in a marriage.

- Thou shalt not postpone joy in a relationship.

- Listening to each other is romantic, because you show that you care enough to listen. That's worth four or five kisses.

- The older you get, the more you intertwine love with respect.

- Watch each other's body language. Care enough to keep a watchful eye and ear.

- There are days when you give 10 or 20 percent, and other days when you give 100 percent.

- It's important to laugh.

- Like each other. You must like what they stand for and who they are.

- People need tender, loving care at any age.

- Hold hands while sitting next to each other when you watch TV. Share love, make love.

- Buy each other beautiful cards and flowers.

- Make life together as full of pizzazz as possible, every single day.

- Ask if you've made it a great day for your partner in little ways.

- Be comfortable with each other, and polish the rough edges.

- Remember, you gain so much from giving.

 

&#10038; **"Nestle up to someone you love and tell them you love them."**

STROKE THRIVER'S GROUP MEMBER

# Glossary

**anomia**
Difficulty in naming objects or retrieving a desired word.

**aphasia**
Difficulty in understanding and using language, resulting from injury to the speech and language areas of the brain. It affects reading, writing, speaking and listening.

**dysarthria**
A speech difficulty that occurs as a result of weakness or paralysis in some or all of the structures used to talk.

**dysphagia**
Difficulty or discomfort in swallowing or inability to swallow.

**homonymous hemianopia** (visual field cut)
A loss of vision in the same visual field in both eyes. This type of partial blindness is usually caused by an injury to the brain.

**verbal apraxia**
A speech difficulty that results in errors in speech production; there is no paralysis responsible for the problem. Apraxic speech, unlike dysarthic speech, is characterized by distortions in sounds and by substitutions or additions of sounds and syllables.

# Resources

## Resources for caregivers

Family Caregiver Alliance
800-445-8106; www.caregiver.org

National Family Caregiver's Association
800-896-3650; www.nfcacares.org

*Today's Caregiver*
800-829-2734; www.caregiver.com

Well Spouse Association
800-838-0879; www.wellspouse.org

## Medical and adaptive equipment

ABLEDATA: 800-227-0216; www.abledata.com

Adaptability catalog (S&S Worldwide): 800-266-8856

AliMed catalog: 800-225-2610; www.alimed.com

Enrichments catalog (Sammons Preston): 800-323-5547

North Coast Medical catalog: 800-821-9319

## Support for stroke survivors

American Stroke Association, a division of the American Heart
   Association
1-888-4STROKE (478-7653); www.StrokeAssociation.org

Sign up for *Stroke Connection Magazine*. Excellent tips for daily self-
   care and many free informational brochures.

Brain Injury Association of America
1-800-444-6443; www.biausa.org

Christopher and Dana Reeve Paralysis Resource Center
www.paralysis.org

Meals on Wheels Association of America
703-548-5558; www.mowaa.org

My Medicine List
www.mnpatientsafety.org
Provides a form you can use to track your medicines.

National Aphasia Association
1-800-922-4622; www.aphasia.org

National Institute of Neurological Disorders and Stroke
www.ninds.nih.gov/disorders/stroke/stroke.htm

National Stroke Association
1-800-STROKES (787-6537); www.stroke.org
Sign up for *Stroke Smart* magazine.

QUITPLAN
1-888-354-PLAN (7526); www.quitplan.quitnet.com
Tobacco Quit Line, providing free counseling over the phone.

# Acknowledgments

A very special thank you to the stroke thrivers and family members who shared their stories. You made this book possible.

**With thanks for generous funding support:** Orlando Helgerson, in memory of Bonnie Helgerson; Steve and Dee Wagner; Lori Boynton and James Helgerson, in honor of Roger Boynton, Sr.; Midwest Coca-Cola Bottling Company; Fairview Foundation; Fairview Press; Pat and Rob Kocsis; David and Tracy Kocsis; John Erickson and Leon Zobel, for both inspiration and financial support.

**Our gratitude to the friends of Fairview Southdale Hospital's Stroke Program and its patients:** Jacquelyn B. Fletcher, for her gift of many hours as co-editor and mentor; Herb Stead, photographer and writer of the first story submitted to this collection; JoAn Blietz and Kevin Jensen, for administrative support; Johanna Rian, Fairview Foundation, for believing in us; Marnee Shepard, PT, NCS, Fairview Southdale Stroke Program manager; Gary Petersen, Director of Cardiovascular Services; Kari Olson, RN, Stroke Program nurse clinician and Unit 55 staff; Nancy Wells, OT, Rehabilitation Director; Jill Sadlowsky, Rehab manager; Fairview Rehabilitation team; Rehabilitation Department support staff; Alexander Zubkov, MD, PhD, co-medical director, Stroke Program; Michael Madison, MD, co-medical director, Stroke Program; Janiece Aldinger, MD, neurologist; Bruce Idelkope, MD, neurologist; Karen Porth, MD, neurologist; Erin Holker, PhD, neuropsychologist, University of Minnesota; Shelli Nelson, RN, cardiac aftercare nurse; Ruth Anne Plourde, MA, Tai Chi instructor; Stephanie Lowrey Whitley, OT; Heather Wessman, OT; Jessica Solie, OT; Ruth Lovander, SLP, Speech-Language Pathology Supervisor; Sheila Clark, SLP; the authors of *Understanding Artery Disease* (Fairview Press); Bachman's Flower and Garden Store, for their lovely setting for our photographs.

**And thanks to all those who serve our community's stroke thrivers:** Fairview Acute Rehabilitation Center staff; Pamela Linnan, Jan Lafavor, Sharon Raasch, and Fairview Ridges Hospital Rehab staff; Judi Johnson and North Memorial Hospital's Stroke Center; Karen Bjorgan and Methodist Hospital's Stroke INSPIRE Program; Sue Newman, Sister Kenny Rehabilitation Center; Courage Center staff; Kathleen Miller and the Minnesota Stroke Association (MSA); Cindy Busch and MSA's aphasia conversation groups; John Mastel, Tess Sierzant, and HealthEast Care System; Minnesota Chapter of the American Stroke Association.

# About the Editors

Candis Fancher, MSCCC, speech-language pathologist, has worked in the field of speech pathology for more than 35 years. She has worked in the hospital setting for 22 years specializing in aphasia therapy. She teaches educational seminars for stroke thrivers on such topics as "Staying Afloat in the Stress Pools of Life," "Embracing Your Changed Brain," and "Integrating Humor into the Healing Process." Candis contributed to the national best-selling book series *Chocolate for a Woman's Soul*. Her love of writing was inspired by her grandfather, and it has become an integral part of the therapeutic process she uses with stroke survivors. She believes that writing helps people discover that their own best therapist lies within. She's been a professional speaker since 1986 and integrates humor into therapy to enhance the healing process.

A source of inspiration for Candis as a young adult was her Grandpa Oliver. As a caretaker for an apartment building, he noticed a pigeon crash against a window and fall into the bushes. Closer observation revealed that the pigeon had broken its leg. While most people would have euthanized the poor suffering "victim," Grandpa had a bright idea: He put a cast on the broken leg and taught "Tumba" how to dance for therapy. Vividly Candis remembers Grandpa clicking his fingers and singing as Tumba danced around in circles, thumping his leg in a rhythmic motion. That pigeon not only walked, he flew to freedom. That's the essence of the healing process: dancing through the pain and discovering the joy of reaching the mountain summit despite the obstacles. Every day, Candis witnesses the joy of self-discovery as each individual's dream becomes a reality and miracles come true.

Lindsey McDivitt has worked to support stroke survivors and their families in rehabilitation centers, communities, and hospitals for more than 25 years. She has edited and written for both regional and national publications, including the American Stroke Association's *Stroke Connection Magazine*. Lindsey has been involved in national stroke initiatives, developing support-group guidelines, peer-visitor programs, conferences, videos and an educational course designed to empower survivors to live well after stroke. She and stroke survivors have greatly benefited from valuable collaborations with the American Stroke Association, National Stroke Association, and other dedicated organizations in our community. In 2005, she was honored by the American Heart Association with the Everyday Hero Professional Award for her contributions to improved quality of life for stroke survivors.Lindsey has a bachelor's degree in Speech and Hearing Science.

JACQUELYN B. FLETCHER is a writer, editor, and marketing professional. Her book *A Career Girl's Guide to Becoming a Stepmom* won a 2008 Parenting Media Excellence Award. She publishes a monthly newsletter that goes out to stepmoms around the world. Since 2001 she's worked as a freelance writer on a vast array of projects, including books, magazines, and websites. She's on the board of directors of the Loft Literary Center in Minneapolis, the largest independent literary center in the country. Find out more about her at www.becomingastepmom.com.

# About the Fairview Southdale Hospital Stroke Program

At Fairview Southdale Hospital, we are passionate about preventing stroke and providing comprehensive, innovative care to save patients' lives and to improve quality of life. As a nationally certified Primary Stroke Center, Fairview Southdale Hospital meets the highest standards of excellence. (Fewer than four percent of hospitals in the country have this certification.) As a Primary Stroke Center, we care for our local community, as well as for patients transferred from other regional hospitals in Minnesota.

### Leading-edge care

Our stroke team of neurologists, interventional neuroradiologists, neurosurgeons, and dedicated staff work together to provide state-of-the-art stroke treatment, rehabilitation, and stroke prevention. The team's expertise and collaborative approach to stroke care helps address all the needs of the stroke patient and the patient's family throughout treatment and recovery.

### Emergency stroke treatment

Medical professionals now have more options for treating stroke early, often preventing or reducing ongoing disabilities. With immediate medical attention and new, innovative techniques, we have the ability to achieve positive outcomes for patients whose condition would have been untreatable in the past.

### Ongoing rehabilitation

At Fairview Southdale Hospital, we realize that rehabilitation is an ongoing journey, and we strive to help people reach their maximum potential throughout all stages of recovery. Our team of physicians, nurses, rehabilitation therapists, registered dieticians, social workers, and chaplains take great pride in providing the specialized care individuals need to return to a satisfying life after stroke. Rehabilitation begins in the hospital during the early days after stroke. This care often continues to acute or subacute settings, as well as to outpatient and home settings. We offer innovative rehabilitation approaches, such as supporting the weight of the body during treadmill training and exercise classes that use Tai Chi to improve balance and flexibility and relieve stress.

### Education and support

Fairview Southdale Hospital offers a variety of aftercare programs to help survivors regain skills and prevent recurrent strokes after they leave the hospital. For more information on these programs, call 952-924-1407, or visit www.fairview.org/climbingthemountain.

### Life in Bloom, an aphasia communication group

Aphasia is a language disorder that can occur from brain damage due to stroke. Exercises can help you as you recover. Life in Bloom is an aphasia communication group designed to inform and inspire you on your way to a better quality of life after stroke. We introduce new strategies for continued rehabilitation of speech and language, brain games, and support.

### Peer visitors

Peer visitors are stroke survivors who have received specialized training in order to provide one-on-one support to other survivors and their families.

### StrokeWise classes

StrokeWise is a series of four classes for stroke survivors and their families that provides an opportunity to learn more about stroke—why it happened, how to prevent it, and how to cope with the aftereffects.

### Stroke Thrivers group

Participate in informative lectures and discussions at your own comfort level, and learn to thrive after a stroke.

### Tai Chi exercise classes

This ancient Chinese "moving meditation" of slow, rhythmic movements focuses on balance, relaxation, and concentration. Tai Chi is a great stress-reliever, and can be done seated. Carepartners, well as survivors, can benefit from the classes.

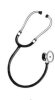

## THE SIGNS AND SYMPTOMS OF STROKE

Even if you've already had a stroke, it's important for you and your loved ones to know the signs and symptoms for stroke. If you experience any of these signs and symptoms, call 911 right away. Keep in mind that these signs and symptoms may go away and then come back. For ways to control of your risk factors, see pages 175–176.

- Sudden numbness or weakness in the face, arm or leg

  (often on one side of the body)

- Sudden confusion or trouble understanding what is going on

- Sudden blurred or decreased vision in one or both eyes

- Sudden difficulty in speaking, understanding speech, or reading

- Sudden trouble with walking, loss of balance, dizziness, or

  problems with coordination

- Sudden, severe headache for no reason

- Fainting or seizures